MW00423281

Advance Praise

"I've been a patient of Dr. Ramaley for over 20 years. He has been a tremendous resource that helped me stay healthy during my career. This is an excellent book with important information that will empower you to improve your health and quality of life."

- Betty Woods, Retired CEO of Premera Blue Cross

"Dr. Ramaley packed so many useful tips into this easy to follow guide on how to improve the quality of our lives and experience more energy. His suggestions are practical, affordable and life-changing. In particular, the summary sheets at the end of each chapter offer specific guidance regarding food, sleep, electronic exposure, exercise and more. While it's written specifically for women, it's a great resource for anyone who wants to experience greater health and wholeness."

- Sheila Colón, Higher Education Consultant

"Fantastic! Fun and easy changes to make for the whole family for a better quality of life!"

- John Herzog, Ph.D., Principle Geologist, GeoEngineers

"As the Executive Director and Founder of Village Volunteers, my life is extremely busy. Dr. David Ramaley has been my primary care doctor for 25 years and I feel very fortunate to have found him. Now that he has written a book, I can share his knowledge with my friends and family around the world to help them gain valuable tools for energy, focus and health. The knowledge in Perpetual Energy has been the key to my productivity, good health, the clarity to juggle many projects and most importantly, attaining balance in life. I have learned to develop a lens that asks the question, "What would Dr. Dave do?" to direct my choices. I highly recommend this book for any busy professional woman."

- Shana Greene, Executive Director of Village Volunteers

Perpetual Energy:
The Ambitious Woman's Quick Guide to More Energy, Focus, and Balance

By Dr. David Ramaley
with Dr. Laurie McQuaig

Seattle Natural Health
Seattle, WA USA

Published 2017

ISBN: 978-1795617956

DISCLAIMER

Cover and book design: Amie Forest
Editing: Laurie McQuaig
Author's photo courtesy of Lindsay Schuette

To my wife Laurie and our two children, Peter and Lise:

you all are my light and energizers in life.

Table of Contents

Introduction

"Look deep into nature and you will understand everything better."

~ Albert Einstein

Perpetual Energy, who doesn't need it? For most people, life is busy. If you are a woman with a demanding career, or with children, or both, you may be checking out this book to see if there is anything you can do to give you more energy, more focus, more vitality. If you are like so many of my patients, you have incessant deadlines, emails to catch up on, PTA meetings, soccer games.... It may feel like a race to get to the end of the next deadline, the next degree, the next promotion, your child's graduation or wedding; all the while you likely still have to make dinner every night, or if you have kids, make sure homework is done, making certain they are safely tucked in, along with all of your other household duties. As a friend used to say about having kids that is applicable to life in general, "The years fly by but the days and nights go on forever." It is in the looking back that you may find perspective. You will likely want to look retrospectively and see that you felt good when you made those deadlines and were still able to go hiking or traveling on the weekends. If you have kids, you will want to look back and see that you had the energy to not only get to all of the games, concerts and meetings, but to also have enjoyed the process and not felt cranky or depressed yourself when your kids were going through their own stages. Kids or no kids, you have a huge task in today's world to stay ahead of it all.

As a holistic doctor for the past 24 years, I have worked with hundreds of professional women ranging from CEOs and business owners to doctors, lawyers, real estate agents, teachers, and mothers who run the PTA. You may be like these ambitious women. You have a sense that there is a higher purpose in life than just yourself, you care about people, family, and relationships; you value your intuition as much as you do your intelligence; you have a keen sense or awareness that the body can heal itself; and you also want to achieve success and reach your goals. You want concrete answers to your problems that can fit into your busy lifestyle.

When I wrote Perpetual Energy, I had you in mind. This book offers a different perspective on health. It comes from years of experience using nature, herbs, vitamins, and lifestyle to treat acute and chronic health conditions. As a naturopath and chiropractor, my scope of practice is similar to an MD's; I can prescribe pharmaceuticals, which at times are necessary, but I always go to nature first. I see how our modern lifestyle has depleted us of our energy, but if we focus on light, water, earth, movement, food, and lifestyle (the chapters of this book), miraculous things can happen, just like they have in my patients' lives. My love for natural healthcare has also come from some very personal experiences that have shaped how I practice today.

When I was 15, I severely hurt my back running on the cross-country team. I could barely walk and was devastated. My mother took me to several doctors and one told me that I would never run again. Intuitively, I knew that this couldn't be right. Finally, my mother took me to a chiropractor that our neighbor had recommended. I barely limped into the clinic, but after one treatment I walked out and soon resumed running again. For me, this was a miracle that I would never forget.

When I was 20, I lived in France after finishing my semester abroad. I applied for an au pair job and went for the interview. The woman had let me know she was a very busy TV producer. She wanted to find the best person to care for her young son. When she opened the door, she greeted me and started to ask me questions. As we were talking I noticed a dark purplish blue line going up her right forearm to her elbow. I asked her if she had hurt her arm, and she said no, but that she had pricked her thumb on a thorn the day before. I said, "Excuse me Madame, I think you need to go to the hospital right away." The interview ended abruptly, and she left for the hospital. She phoned me the next day and said, "You have the job. The doctors said you probably saved my life. I think I can trust you with my son."

Anyone could have made that call; her arm didn't look right. An infection was spreading in her vein toward her heart. This was definitely a case for immediate medical attention, which she received. This experience taught me the importance of observation and intuition, two skills that have served me well in my practice.

In my early 20s, I lived in Central America for a few years working for a human rights organization. I spent most of my time in Nicaragua during the contra war. My wife and I lived in a remote village in the heart of the conflict and saw firsthand the devastation that war inflicts on a people. There was an Argentinian doctor who worked there, and she would often treat many of the wounded civilians. I noticed that she was growing herbs near the clinic for medicinal use. One day I asked her about this, and she said that even though she used drugs and the best of modern medicine to help people survive their injuries, she also wanted to use herbs because that is where the real healing comes from. She further explained that the earth provides us with everything we need, and that despite the killing and brutality she witnessed daily, the earth gave her and the patients she treated a sense of peace, a connection to humanness, a healing that couldn't always be addressed with modern medicine. What an amazing human being she was. She saw the value of modern medicine, but also recognized how we need nature to regain our health. This changed my life and planted seeds for my future career.

These experiences guided me to become a doctor and to realize the value of both alternative and conventional medicine. I am grateful I chose the natural route, because it has given me a different perspective and caused me to delve deeply into finding solutions for my patients' problems. I wouldn't change it for anything.

Over the years, I have studied and researched health issues and written numerous blogs, articles, and patient handouts, but never have I compiled them into one resource. Perpetual Energy is the accumulation of this knowledge and is meant to be a concise, quick guide for the busy woman. What makes it a quick guide is that in most of the chapters you will find Summary and Solutions pages. Feel free to jump to those if you are short on time or want a taste of a chapter. You can always put the book down and come back to a chapter later. Each chapter is independent and can be read in any order. If you make one of these small changes in your health right away, the results will motivate you to keep reading.

*Please note that many of the chapters are peppered with anecdotal case studies of real-life patients. I have changed the names and some of the details to protect privacy, but the actual health history, treatment and results are true. I do not claim this book will solve all of your health issues but it is a beginning. Enjoy the book and the journey.

Chapter 1

Energy

"Energy and persistence conquer all things."

~ Ben Franklin

The secret to perpetual energy begins with a small but powerful particle called the electron. Your body both produces electrons and captures them from your environment in order to power you around the clock. You want to have as many of them in your system as possible. Let me explain. In each atom, there is a nucleus and in each nucleus, there are particles called protons and neutrons. The protons have a positive charge and the neutrons have a neutral charge. Outside of the nucleus, there are tiny electrons that have a negative charge and produce lots of energy. Essentially, your body has (–) electrons and (+) protons, both of which are needed for it to function. However, an excess of electrons produces more energy while protons tend to negate it. This is the holy grail of energy – the more electrons, the more energy produced.

Our current lifestyle compared to that of those who came before us depletes us of electrons and produces too many protons. This book seeks to change this trend by giving you concrete ways to produce and accumulate more electrons in your body. This will help you create more energy in your life and prevent disease.

Running on Fumes

Rachel, a patient, is a great example of how lifestyle can impact energy at any age. At the time she came to see me, Rachel was 29 years old. She was single and the co-chair of computer science at a local college. She worked about 45 hours a week and when she was done with her job she would go home and work on her computer or watch TV. She didn't waste any time telling me that she had lost her mojo. She said that many of her friends were experiencing the same thing and felt like they were running on fumes. Rachel explained that in the past, she and her friends would go out in the evening for drinks or dancing, but no one wanted to do this anymore because they were all too tired. I told her this was unusual for someone her age because humans are designed to be strong and full of energy, particularly at 29.

Back to the science of why Rachel was exhausted, electrons are produced by the mitochondria (the powerhouse) in your cells. These electrons then help create a molecule called ATP that is needed for muscular contraction. Without electrons, all of your muscles would cease to function. This is true of all biological systems in your body. Protons, on the other hand, tend to create inflammation or oxidation. As a matter of fact, every time you sweat, breathe, urinate or defecate your body is naturally getting rid of protons.

To give you an example, molecules called free radicals or oxidants have more protons than electrons. These molecules damage cells and create inflammation, which can lead to heart disease and cancer and cause premature aging. All toxins and infections also create too many protons causing problems in the body. On the other hand, anti-oxidants, like vitamin C, have lots of electrons and they reduce the number of protons thereby lowering the amount of inflammation in the body. The key is to produce more negative electrons and decrease inflammation-producing protons so that we can live longer with less disease and more energy. Let me explain by going back to how our predecessors lived so that you can see how aspects of their way of living kept them healthy.

Think of how they lived, whether as long-ago hunter-gatherers or perhaps as farmers in Nebraska in the mid 1800s. They were outside in light all day, barefoot or wearing leather shoes, gathering or growing all of their own food, drinking fresh water and, most likely, sleeping at least 8-10 hours a night. While their work would have been physically rigorous, they were not exposed to long work hours cooped up in an office with constant mental demands. We now sit for the entire day and evening, eat poor quality foods, avoid the sun and don't get outside as much as we used to. We live under artificial lights, are exposed to toxins and pollutants, use cell phones that emit harmful electromagnetic waves and are surrounded by ubiquitous Wi-Fi. To add to all of this, we have constant phone calls, texts, emails, and deadlines causing us more mental stress. This does not describe a typical day for our ancestors.

As I will explain in the following chapters, our modern lifestyle is robbing us of electrons and producing too many protons. This was Rachel's problem, but fortunately for her, we came up with solutions that increased her electrons and vitality. I will cover these concepts in more detail in the following chapters but essentially this is what I had Rachel do: I sent her outside for light and grounding. We looked at her diet and started her on more nutritious foods and fats. I had her wear blue blocker glasses at work and at night when she was watching TV or was on the computer. It didn't take long for her to get back out dancing and hanging out with friends. She also had more excitement for her job and her life.

Our predecessors lived life immersed in nature. Modern medicine and technological advances have helped us live longer compared to our predecessors who often died younger due to acute infection and trauma. However, on the flip side, we now live with more degenerative disease and fatigue.

You may not want to go back to hunter-gatherer days, but you can adopt many of their practices to create more vitality. This book will revisit those practices and help you implement them. The key is to make frequent contact with nature to obtain energy, while still living and working in a modern technological world.

SUMMARY

- The mitochondria in your cells produce electrons that power your body and give you energy. The more electrons in your body compared to protons, the more energy you have.

- Free radicals contain a lot of protons that cause inflammation, damage your cells, and lead to premature aging.

- The way our predecessors lived produced lots of electrons and most likely resembled how all animals are intended to live.

- Our modern lifestyle and technology tend to rob us of electrons, produce too many protons, and create fatigue.

Chapter 2

Light

"Let there be light."

~ Genesis

"To sit in the shade on a fine day and look upon verdure, is the finest refreshment."

~ Jane Austen

Heidi, a successful 44-year-old mother and lawyer specializing in contract law, is married with two children. She is on the board for a non-profit organization and is also a regular guest lecturer at a university law school. When she came to me, she said that she was suffering from migraine headaches, hair loss, poor concentration and complete exhaustion, as she couldn't sleep through the night. She was alarmed because one of the law partners commented that she didn't seem like herself and that she needed to keep her edge. She was also concerned that she couldn't focus on her family. She described to me her typical day.

She got up early, first going to the kitchen that was lit, like the rest of her home, by LED and fluorescent light bulbs. She immediately looked at her cell phone to check for email and texts. Once her children were up, she fed them and ate a quick breakfast herself before driving them to school. Then at her office, she started working on her computer, sitting under fluorescent lights. She generally took a five to ten-minute mid-morning break. For lunch, she sat at her desk or went to a local restaurant, checking her cell phone often. After lunch, she went back to the office and continued to work on her computer until 5:30. She left work and drove directly to her son's soccer game, where she put on her sunglasses to avoid the sun's glare. She often worked on her computer at night, watching a little TV with the kids, and then helped them with homework and their bedtime routine. She read on her tablet for about 30 minutes before going to sleep.

Does her day seem similar to yours? Her daily routine was triggering her symptoms, depleting her body of energy, and rapidly speeding up the aging process. Let me put her day in the context of our ancestors' world.

Those Who Came Before Us

Our predecessors would have begun their day in natural light, as there was no electricity. Depending on the time of year, they probably spent, on average, 12 hours a day outdoors, and were very aware of the seasons and their environment. Even in the early United States, people were still very connected to light and the seasons as evidenced by the publication of The Farmer's Almanac. First published in 1792, this book was written based on the observation of sunrise and sunset, tides, and other factors.

Our physiology is the same as our predecessors. We still follow a circadian rhythm, meaning that our hormones, brain activity, digestion, sleep patterns, energy production, etc. are all tightly interconnected into a 24-hour cycle. All plants, fungi, animals, and some bacteria thrive around this same 24-hour cycle. If our circadian rhythm goes out of balance, then we will suffer from fatigue and other health problems. Studies show that swing shift workers, who work through the night and sleep during the day, have much higher risks of cancer, diabetes, and heart disease. There is only one way for them to balance their circadian clock – natural light.

The Importance of Light

Natural light consists of a spectrum of wavelengths that are visible and nonvisible (infrared). All forms of light produce energy and heat, with visible light producing smaller amounts of heat and non-visible light producing the most heat. An example of this is when you go outside and see the red in a rose, a form of visible light, but the warmth that you feel on your skin and what warms our planet is non-visible light produced from the sun. Both of these forms are extremely important for producing energy in the body and balancing circadian rhythm. These types of light are absorbed through two portals, your eyes and your skin.

Your eye is an incredible window to the world. There are three ways it functions, and two of these produce energy and balance your circadian rhythm. First, as you know, the eye serves as a camera that takes in visible light and transposes it into images that your brain can understand. Secondly, your eye is a clock that uses visible light to govern your circadian rhythm. It does this through receptors in your eyes called opsins. These receptors don't affect vision, but take in light and send a message to a part of your brain called the hypothalamus. This gland influences "feel-good" neurotransmitters like serotonin and dopamine, as well as hormones in your body affecting metabolism, blood pressure, hunger, and temperature. In addition, the opsin receptors regulate the sleep hormone melatonin, which you may have taken as a supplement for insomnia. The hypothalamus tells the pineal gland to secrete melatonin, but this process is totally dependent on natural light exposure through the eye.

Natural light is so important to your body that you have a gene called clock that exists not only in your eye but also in every single cell of your body. This gene regulates the metabolism and the rest cycle of your cells in a 24-hour period. When light hits the clock gene in your eye, it syncs all of the clock genes in your body to be in harmony. Without natural light, your body will quickly go out of balance.

Thirdly, natural light also stimulates mitochondria electron production in the eye itself, which tells all of the mitochondria in your body to make more energy. This is profound. The very simple act of allowing light into your eye can balance your circadian rhythm, make you feel happy, and produce more energy.

If your eye is a clock, then your skin is a solar panel. Like your eye, it absorbs visible light, but it also absorbs non-visible light or heat. In Chapter 1, I discussed how your mitochondria produce electrons, but what ultimately power the mitochondria are all forms of light. When light hits the skin, it sends a message to the red blood cells (RBC) to come to the skin's surface. When the RBCs arrive, they capture the light and carry it back to the mitochondria where the light can be used to make electrons. Your mitochondria are imploring you, "Bring on the light and sun!" If natural light is so amazing for your vitality, then what might be happening in your life to block it?

The average American spends 97% of the day indoors and stares at computer screens, cell phones, TVs, and tablets for 10.5 hours per day. This means that we are exposed to almost no natural light and have replaced it with what is known as "blue light." This is the type of light we get from all screens like computers, TVs, and cell phones, as well as LED and fluorescent bulbs. There has been a big push to replace all screens and incandescent bulbs with energy-saving LEDs or fluorescent mediums. Although this is good for the environment and decreases our carbon footprint, these newer screens and lights emit an intense narrow wavelength of blue light that enters our eyes and completely disrupts our natural circadian rhythm.

Isolated blue light does not exist in nature because natural blue light is always accompanied by other colors like green and red. Also, the artificial blue light from screens and bulbs is four to six times stronger than natural blue light. Natural blue light, as part of the light spectrum, is strongest in the morning for a short period of time which helps decrease our melatonin and wake us up. However, with the excess of artificial blue light we now take in, we are amped up all day and night. In addition, this form of artificial light produces free radicals that damage the eye, making the mitochondria function poorly. It also adversely affects the hypothalamus and the clock gene, making our hormones and circadian rhythm go out of balance. This can lead to fatigue, weight gain and disease.

How Do We Solve the Problem of Blue Light?

The simplest solution is to wear glasses that block out blue light. Doing this one thing will have a profound impact on your health, energy, and mental clarity. The number of patients who have told me that they feel so much better after wearing blue light blocking glasses is astonishing. Wear these glasses as much as possible when you are looking at a screen or are underneath LED or fluorescent lights, day or night. They are inexpensive and can easily be ordered in non-prescription or magnified readers. I keep an updated list of resources on my website, drramaley.com, that will help you find the most effective glasses. If you wear prescription glasses, ask your optometrist for blue-blocking lenses. If you wear contacts, continue to wear them with a regular pair of blue-blocking glasses. Blue light intensity on screens can be turned down by using apps or in the settings section of your phone or computer. My favorite blue light-blocking app for your computer is called f.lux.

I also recommend that you selectively replace your LED or fluorescent lights with incandescent ones in places in your home or office where you spend a lot of time. If that's not possible, turn off your overhead LED or fluorescent lights and use a lamp with an incandescent bulb. You can continue to use energy-efficient bulbs in areas of your home or office where you spend less time. Currently there are no fluorescent or LED lights that do not create health problems, even if they are full spectrum or daylight color. The old incandescent lights are better, as they come closest to mimicking daylight. In the near future, I believe they will make an energy-efficient light bulb that will be less harmful to your body.

So now that we have blocked out the blue light, bring on the full spectrum natural light! For some of my patients, I actually write on my prescription pad, "Go Outside!" Natural light is free and synchronizes our internal clock to the earth. There is a balance we must strike with the sun in order not to be overexposed but at the same time to get enough full spectrum light, as our ancestors did.

Go Outside

I recommend a minimum of 30 minutes a day of natural light, which can be broken up into segments. Research has shown that even five or ten minutes of natural light will have a positive effect. You do not have to look up at the sky, but merely be outside. You can even be in the shade of a tree or a covered area. The best time to be out in natural light is in the morning. The next best time is midday, especially in summer when the sun is at it's highest. The goal is to get natural light through your eyes and on your skin, but not burn, as this is clearly dangerous. Another thing to consider is that when you wear sunglasses, contacts, prescription glasses, long-sleeved clothes, and lots of sunscreen, you block out the full spectrum of light, losing the benefit of being outside. Your body thinks you are still inside a building.

With natural light exposure, our skin produces a molecule called melanin. Melanin becomes a reservoir of captured light and acts like a battery to power our mitochondria when the light is gone. Melanin also acts as a precursor to melatonin, so the more melanin we have, the better we sleep. Melanin is also a very strong anti-oxidant and protects our skin from damage and cancer. If you are worried about melanoma, the more serious form of skin cancer, The

Lancet, a British medical journal, reported in 2004 that office workers have a higher rate of this form of cancer than people who work outside. This is most likely due to the fact that office workers don't produce enough melanin, as they are cooped up in buildings that do not allow in full spectrum light. For those who have experienced or are worried about skin cancer, I understand your concern. You can modify my recommendations and just expose your arms and legs for a few minutes at a time while wearing a hat to protect your face. Be sure to have regular check-ups with your dermatologist.

Another benefit of sun exposure is the production of vitamin D, which protects you from many cancers and other illnesses. According to Dr. Rathith Nair in the Journal of Pharmacology & Pharmacotherapeutics, vitamin D produced in your skin can last two to three times longer in your body than when you take it orally. To maximize your energy, natural light has to become your best friend. Of course, some geographical areas are much grayer and rainier, but any exposure to natural light is beneficial. Your body and eyes will still capture some of that light energy. I recommend an app called dminder that takes into consideration your skin color, age, gender, where you live, and the hour and day of the month. This app will tell you how much vitamin D you are capturing from the sun and how to avoid burning.

At the beginning of the chapter I wrote about my patient Heidi, who was having a myriad of problems. She changed her habits without much effort and within a month she felt measurably better. She started off by installing the f.lux app to cut down on blue light on her computer, and she adjusted the color temperature to "warm" on her cell phone. She also wore blue blocker glasses. In her home and office, she replaced the lights where she spent the most time with a few incandescent bulbs, maintaining the LED and fluorescent ones for areas with less use. She took an extra few minutes to be in the sun while waiting for her kids after school or when walking from the car to her office building. In fact, she took every opportunity to add a few minutes of light exposure whenever she could. When she went to her son's soccer game, she wore a hat instead of sunglasses to block the sun's glare. She also tried to expose her arms and legs to the natural light. All family members wore blue light-blocking glasses while watching TV. Heidi also made sure to avoid use of any device that emitted blue light for at least 15 minutes before going to bed.

In a recent visit, she told me that her migraines had gone away, she slept through most of the night and felt more alert at work. Most importantly, she said she was more present with her family and had the energy to truly enjoy her kids.

SUMMARY

- All light is energy.

- When light enters the eye, it sets your circadian rhythm and production of energy.

- When light hits your skin, red blood cells come to the surface and carry this light as energy to the mitochondria.

- Light is the most fundamental part of your being, and without it you would wither like a plant in a dark room.

- Sun exposure on your skin creates melanin, which serves as a reservoir of energy to power your battery at night.

- Natural light goes into your eye and directly communicates with the brain and endocrine glands to sync your body with the earth's natural rhythm.

- Vitamin D produced from sun exposure on the skin lasts two to three times longer than when taken orally.

- Modern society has moved us indoors where we now spend 97% of our time. On average, 10.5 hours are spent in front of screens per day.

- Blue light emitted from screens as well as LED and

fluorescent lights are damaging to the eye, disrupting your circadian rhythm and causing fatigue and other health problems.

• When you wear sunglasses, prescription glasses, contacts, or lots of sunscreen outside, your body is tricked into thinking that you are still inside, and you lose the benefits of natural light.

SOLUTIONS

• Go outside, go outside, go outside!

• Go outside for a minimum of 30 minutes a day if possible. This can be broken up into smaller segments of five or ten minutes of natural light, which will have a positive effect on your health.

• To absorb the most natural light, use sunglasses as little as possible when outside. If you use prescription glasses, pull them down on your nose to expose your eyes to as much natural light as possible.

- If you are fair-skinned or prone to skin cancer, go outside for shorter periods of time (five to ten minutes) with just your arms and legs exposed.

- Get as much sun as you can tolerate without burning. When you have had enough, cover up with clothing or use zinc-oxide as sunscreen for protection. Dminder is a good app to help you determine what is a safe level of exposure to the sun and to maximize vitamin D absorption.

- During screen time and while under LED or fluorescent lighting, wear blue-blocking glasses.

- Replace LED and fluorescent lights with incandescent lights in high-use areas of your home and office. To continue to conserve energy, keep energy-saving lights elsewhere in your home and outside. Encourage corporations to create safer light-emitting products.

- Get off your screens at least 15 minutes before bedtime (preferably a lot longer).

Chapter 3

Earth

"Of all the paths you take in life, make sure some of them are dirt."

~ John Muir

"I'm barefoot whenever I can be."

~ Shakira

About 15 years ago Brianna, a 29-year-old architect, came to see me. She was experiencing numbness and tingling in her feet and hands. Her symptoms had been present for about a year and were getting worse. She also noticed that when she walked, she had difficulty keeping her balance and could not fully feel her feet as they hit the ground. I had seen patients with these symptoms before and usually a couple of chiropractic adjustments would resolve the symptoms. After a few treatments, however, she wasn't getting better and I changed course. I sent her out for an MRI of her brain and spine and the films revealed she had some white lesions in her brain indicating Multiple Sclerosis. I referred her to a neurologist and the diagnosis was confirmed.

The neurologist wanted her to start several medications immediately, but Brianna wanted to try other approaches first. She was extremely depressed about the diagnosis, as she was a very active woman who loved hiking and physical exercise. She started to cry, saying she couldn't bear the thought of a life limited by MS. She asked me for advice. I had currently been studying the effects of "grounding," or going barefoot on the earth, as treatment for numerous neurological and autoimmune diseases. I myself had been doing this for several years to cure a decade-long knee injury that had prevented me from running. This treatment had completely eased my pain and given me back my life as a runner. I told Brianna about my own experience and the scientific studies I had read about grounding. I suggested that she do some grounding to see if it might lessen some of her symptoms. Since she was highly motivated, she took this to heart, and the next day she spent four hours outdoors barefoot, grounding to earth. She even wore shorts and a tank top and lay flat on the grass to get as much contact as possible. After faithfully following this routine for a month, she came back to report her symptoms were essentially gone – and to this day, her symptoms are manageable.

Grounding may not resolve a serious illness completely, but it can be used in conjunction with other treatment and be of great benefit.

How Can Grounding Help Someone Diagnosed With MS?

In Chapter 1, I discussed that virtually all energy in the body comes from the electrons that the mitochondria produce. The opposite of the electron is the proton, which tends to produce inflammation and disease. I wanted Brianna to get as many electrons into her body as possible to help lower her inflammatory state. According to Dr. Feynman, a well-known physicist from California Institute of Technology (Caltech), the earth is likely our greatest reservoir of electrons. We don't know why the earth produces so many electrons, but most likely it is from the daily lightning strikes that happen around the world approximately eight million times per day or from the sun's energy hitting the earth's surface.

Our ancestors were connected to the earth. They went barefoot or wore moccasins or some type of all leather or natural fiber footwear. Compare this to today, where we spend our days on carpet and synthetic floors wearing shoes and sandals made with rubber soles. When was the last time you placed your bare feet on a patch of grass, dirt, or sand? To get the benefit of earth's electrons, we cannot have any synthetic substance or wood in between our skin and the earth.

According to cardiologist Steven T. Sinatra, M.D., disconnection from the earth is one reason we feel tired. Think back again to a time when you were barefoot at the beach. Do you remember putting your feet in the sand? How about walking barefoot along the ocean's edge and feeling energized? This is not just a placebo effect; it is the actual influx of electrons into your body giving you more energy.

Rates of inflammatory and autoimmune disease have skyrocketed in the last 40 years. Research has demonstrated that grounding can reduce the stress hormone cortisol, improving blood pressure and decreasing inflammatory markers. Think of the impact grounding can have on autoimmune diseases that are the result of inflammation. Even with injuries, no matter how serious, grounding can have a profound impact.

Several years ago, I was running and tripped in a hole. The second this happened I felt a searing pain in my lower right leg and fell to the ground. I knew immediately I had not merely sprained my ankle but had torn muscles and tendons. I hopped back to my car, over a mile away, and felt like I was going into shock. An MRI revealed that I had near complete tears of my gastrocnemius and soleus muscles. With these types of injuries, there is severe swelling and blood pooling, creating a deep purple color in the skin. My doctor told me to be prepared for a long recovery period. He told me it would take many weeks or even months to heal. I knew that grounding had helped my knee in the past, so in addition to herbs and other natural modalities, I went to a park and lay on the grass with the back of my leg contacting the earth. I did this daily. Within two weeks, I was no longer using my crutches. In about six weeks, I was able to start running short distances. This was easily half the normal recovery time. After this experience, I made it part of my weekly routine to ground myself, which also increased my energy and helped me sleep more soundly.

Grounding in a High-Tech World

Clearly, the vast majority of us aren't going to go barefoot all day. There are, however, some very practical things that you can do, even in an urban environment. First, find a conductive surface like grass, dirt, rock, sand, or cement (which is made from shale and rock). Any of these mediums will conduct electrons from the earth. Even walking on your cement sidewalk or cement garage floor barefoot will ground you. Asphalt, made from petroleum products, cannot ground you. Most streets are made of asphalt, so stick to the sidewalk. Going barefoot inside your home won't ground you because carpets, wood floors, and other flooring materials are synthetic surfaces. Secondly, try to wear all leather shoes. I have posted on my website several companies that make all-leather shoes or sandals. Thirdly, weed your garden or lawn with bare hands and make contact with grass or dirt – this is a great way to ground.

The amount of time you need to ground depends on your stress level, toxins, and amount of inflammation in your body. At a minimum, I suggest 10 minutes a day, as this is probably realistic for most people. You can stay out longer when weather and time permit. There is no such thing as grounding for too long. I work in an urban area and find patches of grass, dirt, or cement to stand on in all leather shoes during a coffee break or lunch. This can be for just a five-minute break, but your body will love it. Get creative and make it a game. People keep track of their steps per day; why not keep track of grounding time? Use this time to do some deep breathing or just be present. Turn off your cell phone, or put it on airplane mode and look at the sky, the trees, and the birds. I have heard from many patients that when they do this, even for just a brief period, they feel recharged, alert, and more productive.

As for Brianna, I still see her as a patient 15 years later. She follows up periodically with her neurologist, and he confirms she is doing well. She is in great health, she maintains a healthy diet, takes some supplements, and is the most avid grounder I have ever known. She still gets some occasional numbness and tingling, and when this happens she grounds more and her symptoms tend to go away. In a recent visit, she complained of slight foot pain, so I asked her to take off her sock to examine her foot. When she did this, I noticed several blades of grass stuck between her toes, and she laughed and explained that she had just finished walking barefoot in the park. I couldn't have been happier. I have watched this amazing human being transform her health by connecting to the earth, like our ancestors have done for thousands of years.

SUMMARY

- The earth is a reservoir of negative electrons.

- Too many protons cause inflammation and electrons reduce inflammation.

- Going barefoot on the earth facilitates the flow of electrons into the body, thereby lowering inflammation and increasing energy. Leather-soled shoes permit the flow of electrons as well.

- To get the benefit of earth's electrons, we must be on grass, dirt, sand, or concrete. Synthetic flooring substances, asphalt, or wood block the flow of electrons as does wearing rubber-soled shoes.

- Research has demonstrated that grounding lowers elevated cortisol.

SOLUTIONS

- Ground for a minimum of ten minutes a day, but more is better.

- You can ground by standing barefoot on dirt, sitting barelegged on the grass, lying on the beach, or by getting your hands in the dirt in your garden. You can even ground by standing barefoot on your cement garage floor.

- It is possible to buy grounding mats and bed sheets. Check out drramaley.com for information and links.

Chapter 4

Food

"Don't eat anything your great- grandmother wouldn't recognize as food."

~ Michael Pollan

Nikki is a professor at a local university. She has two children, 9 and 11, and is married. She has an excellent job and tries her best to take good care of her children. She came to see me with her children because the whole family kept getting sick. They each had a runny nose, and when one person in the family got ill, they all got ill. She frequently had to call in sick to work, and was falling behind in her responsibilities. Both she and her kids were gaining weight, and Nikki complained of chronic chest pain and a cough that wouldn't go away. She had seen two doctors who prescribed numerous antibiotics, but they didn't help her. One of her children already had tubes put in his ears. She was frustrated. After I listened to more of Nikki's history, she told me that she wondered if the family's poor health was related to the food they were eating. She had been so busy lately and had been less attentive to their diet. She had been resorting to convenience foods to serve her family. I asked her, "Are you ready to try something fun with your kids?" For many years, I've taken groups of patients on a tour of our local farmers market. I invited her and her children to join the group. They were game, so we made a plan. That Saturday, her whole family showed up. That day changed their lives for the better.

Food is a Key to Unlocking Your Genetic Code

In my farmers market tours, I want people to understand that food is not just fuel for the body, but a key to unlocking our genetic code. An example of this is a profound study that was done several years ago on Agouti mice. These mice have yellow fur and are genetically prone to obesity, cancer and diabetes. Researchers wanted to see if dietary changes for the mice could have any effect on their offspring. They fed them foods high in B12, folic acid, betaine, and choline (methyl groups). The results were significant. The offspring were born with brown fur, were lean, and were less prone to cancer and diabetes. In other words, the DNA of the lean and non-diabetic offspring was identical to the obese mother's DNA, but the unhealthy genes never got triggered or expressed. The mother's diet actually switched off those genes so the offspring were healthy. This study perfectly illustrates a concept called epigenetics. Epigenetics is completely rewriting our understanding of genes, disease, and health. The essence of this is simple: For genes to express themselves as cancer, diabetes, obesity, or fatigue, those genes have to be turned on, or else they just lie dormant. The key is to not trigger those specific genes and instead to turn on healthy genes.

When we eat food, it gets broken down and releases all sorts of phytochemicals and molecules that as I said above, go beyond just providing nutritional content. Literally, these compounds tell our genes what to do. They are the conductor of our genome. Research shows that the more colorful and complex the food, the greater the genetic expression for health. For the most complex plants to grow, they need to be in a complex environment.

Let's pretend you are a conventionally grown broccoli. You grow in soil that is devoid of nutrients, fungi, and bacteria. You have been sprayed with pesticides numerous times during your life. Essentially, there are no predators, so you become lazy and think, "I can just chill here and do nothing." You become a couch potato or, I should say, a "couch broccoli."

Now think of yourself as a broccoli grown organically by a local farmer. You spend your day in soil with lots of beneficial bugs and fungi, and you haven't been sprayed with petrochemicals. You have to fend for yourself, so when that cutworm or aphid comes around to eat you, you do whatever it takes to stay alive. You take the nutrients from the rich organic soil, and you produce large amounts of anti-oxidants called sulforaphanes, glucosinolates, and many more phytochemicals we don't even know about yet. These phytochemicals repel the predators, and you stay alive.

This event creates different gene expression (epigenetics) in the plant that will help it to be stronger and more resistant to disease and illness. These rich molecules are also what produce the color of the plant so, generally speaking, the richer and more varied in color, the more beneficial information the plant has. In essence when we eat these plants, we inherit or absorb their genetic information, so we in turn can express better health. This process has been going on for thousands of years. It is almost as if the plants are becoming part of us. Do you want to eat a couch broccoli or a broccoli that is super-fit and robust?

Our ancestors ate wild, foraged, or cultivated plants without pesticides. Depending on where they lived, they probably ate well over 200 different types of foods of all colors and shapes, as well as numerous types of wild and domesticated animals. Since 1900, we have lost a majority of the variety of foods eaten in the US. Today, the average American eats just 30 different types of foods in a year. We also use over one billion pounds of pesticides every year. Let's go back to the tour and see what Nikki learned about how farmers markets resist these trends.

At the Market

First, we stop at a vegetable stand and look at potatoes. There are ten different varieties, some with blue, red, purple, and dark yellow colors. They have names like Purple Viking, Mountain Rose, Red Lasoda, All Blues, and Purple Majesty. The deep colors mean lots of phytochemicals and anti-oxidants are present. The potatoes even have some blemishes on them where an aphid or beetle tried to attack. There's lots of genetic information in those potatoes! There are over 700 varieties of potatoes in the world, but we generally eat just one – the Russet. Nikki's kids pick out the Purple Majesty and All Blues, and in the basket they go. Next we see cauliflower; it is a brilliant purple and yellow. Yes, purple and yellow. There is a beautiful Romanesco broccoli. It is chartreuse in color, is a complete fractal and is full of spirals. Think of the genetic information in that vegetable! The Romanesco goes in their basket.

The mushroom stand next door has all sorts of varieties including chanterelle, wild oyster, and lobster that are yellow, orange, and black. They contain so much more information than just the common button mushroom that we are used to eating. They also don't go through photosynthesis like most plants, and instead feed on decaying matter, which gives them entirely different genetic information than other plants. They are also prone to predators like the slug and certain bacteria, so we get the benefit of the phytochemicals that protect them. There are so many edible plants that I could talk about at the market, but the kids are getting tired, so we move on to one of the most important aspect of the farmers market – the animal products.

There is no other way to put this but to simply state that the animals we eat in the US are sick. This is not an over-exaggeration. 99% of our chickens, pigs, beef, and turkey are raised in feedlots, fed genetically modified soy and corn, growth hormones, numerous pharmaceuticals, antibiotics, arsenic, and who knows what else. Feedlots use a lot of resources and pollute our streams and rivers with manure. The vast majority of these animals are treated inhumanely and never see daylight. Most of the cattle develop colitis and infections of the stomach. Close to 70% of the chickens in the US contain arsenic. If you eat sick animals, you will be a sick animal. Period.

On the other hand, if you eat animals that were raised humanely – allowed to forage on grass, plants and bugs – you can be just as healthy as they are. When was the last time you saw an animal in the wild eating lots of corn and soy?

When we visit the next stand, there is a beautiful selection of meat and dairy. All of these products are from animals raised on grass and allowed to go outdoors. The owners of the farm tell us they consider themselves grass farmers more than ranchers, because the health of the herd is completely tied to the health of the soil, grass, and plants. If the animals eat healthfully, they will be healthy. She tells us they have almost no veterinarian bills and don't have to use antibiotics because the animals rarely get sick. Nikki's ears really perk up at that explanation, and I'm sure she must be thinking of her own kids' health. The owner grabs a steak and shows us how the fat is yellow, not white like conventional beef, since the fat is full of beta-carotene from the grass. As a consumer, the advantage of grass-fed animals over feedlot animals is twofold: One, they have a much lower level of unhealthy pro-inflammatory omega-6 fats compared to the healthy anti-inflammatory omega-3 fats. Animals that are fed corn and soy convert these grains to omega-6 fats whereas animals that are grass-fed convert the grass to omega-3 fats. Our ancestors, who ate wild nongrain fed animals and wild fish, probably had about a 2:1 or at the most a 4:1 ratio of omega-6 to omega-3 profile. Today, the average American has an approximate 20:1 ratio, causing lots of inflammation. Most grass-fed animals will eat anywhere from six to 15 different types of grass and plants and chickens will eat an assortment of bugs. This gets turned into information to help with our own genetic expression.

The Environment and Grass-Fed Animals

From an environmental point of view, grass-fed animal farming has been endorsed by the Sierra Club and the Union of Concerned Scientists as a sustainable practice. The grasses actually capture carbon and sequester it in the soil. Nikki adds some hamburger, bacon, and two dozen eggs. She also buys milk, cheese, and yogurt there, as it has a nice rich yellow color to it from all of the carotenoids. The kids seem super excited, and when the owner shows them pictures of the cows on their farm, they can see the animals really are on grass fields chewing their cud.

I followed up with Nikki about two months after the tour and she said that her cough, weight problem, and sickness had cleared up, and her kids were much healthier. She reported that she couldn't get to the farmers market all the time, but once she got the concept about color, grass, and genetics, she found it easier to go to grocery stores and make better choices.

Now you may be thinking to yourself that this is all good, but how do I afford this and how do I get a hold of this food with my busy lifestyle? First of all, make it a priority. We spend about 90% of our food budget on processed food. The average American in 1960 spent 18% of their income on food and 6% on medical bills. Today, it is almost 19% on medical bills and 6% on food. Do you see something happening here? "Your food is your best medicine" is not just a saying, it is the absolute truth.

So here are some very simple rules. Buy color and lots of it. Buy organic whenever you can and, when possible, either grow your own food or go to the farmers market. Buy organic, grass-fed meats, eggs, and dairy products. It is also possible to buy meat and some dairy products and freeze them to avoid having to make extra trips. I shop many of our conventional grocery stores to check out prices, and the cost difference between grass-fed and non-grass-fed meat is not as great as it was before.

I still see Nikki and her kids at the farmers market and they are very healthy. Nikki tells me that they rarely have to see a doctor. I can't help but peek in her basket and what a beautiful sight it is; lots of lush dark greens and bright red, yellow, and blue vegetables. My job here is done.

SUMMARY

- Food turns on and off your genetic code. The more color and variety in your food, the greater the expression of healthy genes.

- The more stress a plant has, the more phytochemicals it produces. Phytochemicals act as anti-oxidants and they help turn on and off genes for optimal health. This is why organic produce is better.

- Our ancestors most likely ate over 200 varieties of foods depending on where they lived. Americans today eat on average only 30 different types.

- Grass-fed animals are healthier and contain more omega-3 oils, beta-carotene, and vitamin E.

- Grass-fed farming has been endorsed by the Sierra Club and the Union of Concerned Scientists as a sustainable practice that doesn't contribute to global warming.

- The average American in 1960 spent 18% of their income on food and 6% on medical bills. Today, it is almost 19% on medical bills and 6% on food.

- Food can determine how your genes are turned on and off to express optimal health. This is called epigenetics.

- Your food can determine how your jeans fit.

SOLUTIONS

- Eat a rainbow of colors in your diet, preferably locally and organically grown.

- Try to eat mostly grass-fed meats, eggs and dairy products.

- Don't be afraid to try different foods that you haven't eaten before because the more variety of food you eat, the greater genetic information your body takes in.

- Eat fermented foods like unpasteurized sauerkraut, kefir, and kombucha. These are great sources of probiotics.

- Excellent food related resources include: eatwild.com, the Weston A. Price Foundation (westonaprice.org), or Michael Pollan's Food Rules: An Eater's Manual, to name a few.

Chapter 5

Fats

"With enough butter, anything is good."

~ Julia Child

Yes, you read that quote right. Foods do taste better with butter, and it is good to eat some now and again. Anthropological studies show that our ancestors ate plenty of fat, mostly from animal sources including fish. Calorie for calorie, fat gives you the most energy. If you remember in Chapter 1, mitochondria make ATP and electrons that translate into energy. We want to eat foods that make the most energy. Consider that one molecule of sugar produces 38 ATP, whereas one molecule of fat produces about 138 ATP. Fat is an amazing source of energy. As a matter of fact, your body can survive on a diet made up almost entirely of fat and some protein without ever consuming sugar and carbohydrates. Your body can convert fat into glucose as well as ketones that the brain can use as a fuel source. We humans are efficient fat burners. We most likely developed this attribute over thousands of years of using our own fat as fuel, which allowed us to travel great distances or go for long periods of time without food.

If you have reservations about eating fat, realize that in 1900 the average American consumed 35-40% of calories from fat. This included 20 pounds of butter per year (today we eat four), plus eggs, lard, and cream. History shows that they had lower rates of cancer, heart disease and diabetes. If we exclude childhood mortality, trauma, and infection, on average, they lived almost as long as we do today.

Traditionally, the Inuit Native Americans in Alaska ate a diet almost exclusively of fat. The average mid-Victorian living in England in the 1850s ate close to 35% of their calories as fat, mostly from beef, lamb, and lots of fish and shellfish. The animal fats that these various groups ate came from pasture-fed animals that ate a wide variety of grasses and from marine animals that ate a variety of fish. This biodiversity in the animals' diets produced a large spectrum of genetic information, just like plants in your garden or those from the farmers market. Today, the average French person consumes four times as much butter and 60% more full fat cheese than an American, yet they have less heart disease. While I am not advocating that everyone eat copious amounts of fat, just realize that fat is not your enemy, and can help you increase your energy.

A Good Fat Bad Fat Story

An example of a patient who needed to eat more fat is Janelle. When she came to see me, she was frustrated, upset and in tears. She said her energy had been declining the last three years, but in recent months, she felt so tired that she wanted to sleep all day. Her sister had just been diagnosed with breast cancer and this made her think of her own health and mortality. She was a well-known psychiatrist and had lots of stress because she recently expanded her clinic with more staff and doctors. Her 18-year-old son was depressed and she couldn't stop worrying about him. She also thought she was developing a neurological disease because she had a burning sensation on her skin, but there were no rashes or lesions. She said she experienced brain fog, was easily distracted, and often had a hard time processing conversations. This terrified her because of the nature of her work. She was gaining weight, her clothes no longer fit, her libido was waning, and she felt winded even going up a flight of stairs.

As I delved more into her history, things became clearer.

About four years before, she went to a routine physical and her labs revealed a slightly elevated cholesterol level. The doctor thought that because Janelle's mother had died from a stroke at age 72, Janelle should follow a low-fat diet and take a statin, a cholesterol lowering medication. Although Janelle felt fine at the time, she thought it wasn't a bad idea since she was trying to lose about ten pounds and she believed that cutting back on fat might benefit her and her whole family. She looked online for more information and found a few books on low-fat cooking. She adopted the low-fat lifestyle, eliminated the foods that were high in saturated fats, and replaced them with vegetable oils like canola, corn, soy, and safflower. She started on 20 mg of a statin and seemed fine with this new medication. About a year later after she had made these changes, she started to develop symptoms.

I looked at her most recent lab work and saw why she was not well. Her cholesterol level was 143, too low for a 44-year-old female. Although this may seem contrary to popular opinion, cholesterol and fat are absolutely necessary for your body to function. Not only was Janelle deficient in fat, but also the fats she was consuming were the wrong types, depriving her body of energy.

As Janelle learned, her low-fat diet and medication were robbing her body of precious cholesterol, omega-3 oils and saturated fats. She was replacing them with highly refined inflammatory vegetable oils called omega-6 fats, primarily from canola, corn, soy, and safflower that had until recently never been consumed by humans. Here is how this seems to have come about.

In the early 1950s, as the advent of processed food and food additives boomed, the theory of heart disease was formed. Cholesterol and saturated fats were blamed for heart disease, which eventually dealt a deathblow to butter, eggs, red meat, and many dairy foods. Substitute butter, called margarine, was introduced and a whole industry began, propagated by processed food companies and leading to the low-fat diet craze of the 60s and thereafter. Today, the low-fat diet phenomenon produces about $60 billion a year in consumer spending. We have experienced an exponential increase in heart disease, cancer, diabetes, Alzheimer's, and many other illnesses and this may be due in part to these societal and dietary changes.

Why You Need Fat

Cholesterol and saturated fats play a key role in your health. For example, every cell in your body has a membrane that acts as a protective barrier between the inside and outside of the cell. This membrane allows the cell to breathe, take in nutrients and eliminate waste. The membrane consists of nearly 50% cholesterol, and without the proper amount of cholesterol, the cell ceases to function effectively. Interestingly, you also need fat and cholesterol for your nervous system. Your nerves are enveloped by something called myelin, which acts like an insulating plastic coating around an electrical cord. Myelin is mainly composed of cholesterol and some water. If you lose myelin, the nerves won't conduct well and will slow down their transmission. There are numerous symptoms and diseases that occur with poor nerve conduction, the most well-known being Multiple Sclerosis. In addition to your nerves and cells needing cholesterol, the brain uses lots of it also. The brain contains 25% of your body's total cholesterol and has its own mechanism for producing it since it is so important to its function. In a study cited in the British Journal of Psychiatry, June 1993, it concluded that the lower the cholesterol levels, the greater the risk of depression and suicide, especially as you age.

Another important function of cholesterol is to make sex hormones such as estrogen, progesterone, testosterone, cortisol, and DHEA. These hormones keep you looking young and thin and help you produce energy. I often see patients who have taken statins to lower their cholesterol and whose sex hormones have plummeted, causing them to feel fatigue, lose libido, have brain fog, and gain weight. This was the case with Janelle. Not only was she taking statins, but she was also on a low-fat diet, limiting her production of cholesterol and decreasing her sex hormone production. There are times when statins are beneficial, but they are often overprescribed.

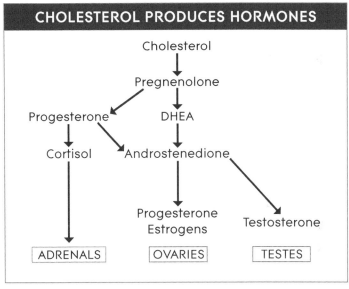

CHOLESTEROL PRODUCES HORMONES

As you can see in the diagram, your main hormones are made from cholesterol.

Some of you may be concerned that if you don't have low cholesterol you will be more prone to heart disease. Current research is showing that the main culprit of heart disease is inflammation and not necessarily elevated cholesterol. If you remember from the previous chapter, omega-6 oils are largely responsible for the production of inflammation and omega-3 oils are anti-inflammatory. When Janelle switched to a low-fat diet and replaced saturated fat with omega-6 vegetable oils, she was replacing omega-3 fats with omega-6 fats. While you need some omega-6 fats, you may be over-consuming them. Your body was not designed to process so many omega-6 fats. Your ancestors probably had a ratio of 4:1 or even 2:1 of omega-6 to omega-3 fats. Today, most Americans are at 20:1 or higher. There is now a test that measures the ratio of omega-6 to omega-3 fats. This test is a good indicator of your overall health. Check my website, drramaley.com for more information about this test.

To increase your omega-3 fats, consume more seafood, grass-fed meats and fish oil. To decrease your omega-6s, stay away from the processed food and bakery aisles. Non-grass-fed cows eat corn and soy, producing meat and dairy products high in omega-6 oils. Corn, soy and canola oils also contain omega-6s.

Back to Janelle: She threw out all of her vegetable oils, but saved her olive, coconut, and avocado oils because these are lower in omega-6 fats. I told her to bake with butter or coconut oil. I encouraged her to buy grass-fed butter and meat, whole milk, and a healthy array of vegetables. I also gave her a list of grocery items that contain good fats and oils, such as crackers made with olive oil or butter. Once she started looking, she found plenty of options for healthy meals and snacks. She began eating a moderate amount of grass-fed meat and bacon and didn't hesitate on her butter, coconut, and avocado consumption. At least twice a week, she ate wild fish with high omega-3 fats while avoiding farm-raised fish, which have the same high omega-6 composition as factory-fed animals. I also gradually took her off the statin, as it was contributing to her symptoms as well. A month after she made her dietary changes, her energy came back. She felt so much better, was having sex again, had lost weight, and her brain fog had cleared up. Her teenage son also benefitted from the new diet and his depression improved. Janelle's cholesterol went up to 202, which is still within the healthy range. Her inflammatory marker (hs-CRP), which had been moderately high when I first saw her, came into the normal range after these lifestyle changes.

I recommend that you enjoy healthy fats, which will most likely cause you to lose weight and have more energy. In the words of one of my heroes, Julia Child, "If you're afraid of butter, use cream."

SUMMARY

- Fat is a rich source of energy; it produces 138 ATP whereas sugar or carbohydrates produce 38 ATP per molecule.

- The average American in 1900 consumed 35–40% of calories from fat.

- The French consume four times as much butter and 60% more full fat cheese than Americans and have less heart disease.

- Your body needs cholesterol to be healthy. Almost all hormones are produced from cholesterol. The brain contains 25% of your body's total cholesterol and your cell membranes are 50% cholesterol.

- Omega-3s are mainly anti-inflammatory and omega-6s are pro-inflammatory. It is thought that our ancestors' ratio of these two fats was approximately 4:1 or 2:1, whereas Americans today have, on average, have a ratio of 20:1. This imbalance creates inflammation and disease.

- Omega-6s are found in almost all processed foods and conventionally raised (non-organic, grain-fed) animal products.

SOLUTIONS

- Consume omega-3 oils, including all wild fish (salmon, halibut, sardines, and cod have the highest amounts), hemp and flaxseed oils. Other oils with healthy fat ratios are avocado, coconut and olive.

- Avoid soy, corn, canola, safflower and cottonseed oils.

- Eat some foods with cholesterol and saturated fats, like eggs, butter, full-fat cheese and yogurt, preferably from grass-fed animals.

- Try to avoid statin medications and use only if absolutely necessary, as the side effects can create fatigue and muscle pain.

Chapter 6

Water

"Water is the driving force of all nature."

~ Leonardo da Vinci

Imagine drinking water several hundred years ago. It was probably from a stream, river, or spring. The water was pure, moving, cool, and ran over rocks or other objects that created a swirling or spiral motion. There was no chlorine, fluoride, or pollutants.

Clearly there are many benefits to today's drinkable water as it has greatly diminished rates of waterborne illness and disease. However, water has been reduced to a utilitarian substance without appreciation for its true impact on health and human expression. For example, if you drink tap water, it quenches your thirst and keeps you alive, but research by water experts is showing that spring water has more to offer. Science is just beginning to prove what our ancestors may have known, that water is more than just a molecule, it truly is life and forms who we are as humans.

The Dehydrated Executive

Lisa, a 58-year-old marketing executive, came to me complaining of right shoulder pain and also said she felt really stiff and could barely move. She had spent a lot of time and money seeing different doctors to find out why she was in so much pain. She was finally diagnosed with frozen shoulder syndrome, but the medications weren't alleviating her symptoms and the rest of her body still hurt. She said she felt very old and noticed that her patience with clients was getting short. Her main stress reliever was her Pilates class, but she could no longer go to it because of the pain.

Straight away, I observed that her skin completely lacked elasticity and fullness. I asked if she had been drinking water and she said yes, about three glasses of tap water a day. I then conducted a simple diagnostic test I call the Ramaley Dehydration Test (see drramaley.com). I asked her to sit with her right arm relaxed by her side. I told her that I would slowly lift her arm in an arc motion, and that she should tell me when it started to hurt. As I lifted her arm to ten degrees, she said it hurt terribly; a normal range of motion for a shoulder should be 180 degrees. Next, I brought in four glasses of water: tap, filtered, spring, and EZ water (I'll explain this later). I had her drink the tap water and there was no difference in her range of motion. She then drank filtered water and she got about a 30-degree increase in her range before the pain began, a good improvement. Next, she drank spring water. After drinking this, she was able to raise her arm pain-free to 140 degrees. She then drank spring water that had been "structured" (EZ water) and, even more impressive, her arm went up to 160 degrees without pain. This was quite amazing considering she was diagnosed with a frozen shoulder. I explained to her that she was extremely dehydrated and when she drank good water, her body responded immediately. Even though she was drinking three glasses of tap water a day, it was not enough and it was poor quality water. It really didn't meet her hydration requirements. I will explain in this chapter how Lisa eliminated her pain and increased her energy, and how vibrant water may help you to relieve pain that is keeping you from doing your job or being active.

Imagine your body is like a battery, and there is little to no water in it. You may have heard that sound of an almost-dead battery trying to turn an engine over. This is what your body is like without enough good water: barely functioning. The average American drinks 2.5 – 3.8 glasses of water a day and urinates about 6.5 glasses of liquid. You do the math. Do you wonder why your skin isn't vibrant and you feel so stiff? Most medical books say we are about 60% water, and while this is true by weight and volume, water makes up 99% of all of our molecules. We literally are water and how much, and the type we drink, becomes the expression of who we are. Albert Szent-Gyorgi, the famous physiologist and Nobel Prize winner for the discovery of vitamin C said, "Water is life's matter and matrix, mother and medium. There is no life without water."

So, if you are 99% water, then clearly you want to drink water that is as pure and natural as possible. In Lisa's case, tap water made only a slight difference in her shoulder range of motion because it contained chlorine, fluoride and pollutants. These chemicals can inhibit how water enters our cells so that even though we are drinking water, we remain dehydrated. Filtering water takes out these toxic substances, allowing your body to utilize it more effectively. Even better is spring water. Scientists have demonstrated that water that is fast-moving, pressurized and cool in temperature, contains more electrons. Spring water has these exact attributes because it comes from deep in the earth. The increased amount of electrons in spring water may explain why it helps people regain their health and why it tastes so good. This is perhaps why Lisa's shoulder range of motion improved so much. Personally, I have noticed the popularity of drinking spring water grow as there are more people at the spring where I get my water. It has now become the "local watering hole," busy all the time with lots of conversation about water. Spring water is also the best medium for producing EZ water in your body and this was the water that Lisa drank last and saw the most improvement from. I believe EZ water has many health benefits and great potential for future research.

Water the EZ Way

In his book, The Fourth Phase of Water, University of Washington professor Dr. Gerald Pollack redefines our perception of water. He says there is a fourth phase of water that is not gas, solid, or liquid as we know it, but is what he calls Exclusion Zone (EZ) water or Structured Water. He says that EZ water is different than regular water. Regular water, or what we may see come out of the tap, contains electrons and protons as well as other substances from the environment. EZ water, on the other hand, contains just negative electrons and almost nothing else. Did you catch that? Electrons. Remember, a high concentration of electrons produces lots of energy.

What other doctors and scientists have theorized using Pollack's research is that EZ water is crucial to the functioning of the systems in your body, making your cells work better, blood flow more easily, muscles contract more strongly, and DNA replicate properly. The most important part though is that EZ water is made up of negative electrons, the holy grail of energy. These theories pertaining specifically to the body can be complicated and I cannot cover them completely in this book. For further information go to my website drramaley.com for direct links to see interviews with Dr. Pollack about research he has done. The takeaway about electron-rich EZ water is this: the more you have, the better and the more energetic you will feel. The cool thing about EZ water is that, while a slight oversimplification, it already exists inside of you, you just need to make more of it. And to make more of it, guess what you need? Light, earth and good water. Let me explain.

In his lab, Dr. Pollack demonstrated healthy light makes EZ water. He put an open-ended tube in water and then shined light over the water and negatively charged EZ water started forming and flowing through the inside of the tube. Pollack also found that when exposed to infrared or visible light, humans became more negatively charged too, meaning more electrons were present. Thomas Cowan, M.D., in his book, Human Heart, Cosmic Heart, builds on Pollack's research by hypothesizing that when light makes

EZ water in the body, like the tube in Pollack's experiment, this process aids the flow of blood in addition to the pumping action of the heart. This theoretical increase in blood flow means that you get more oxygen and nutrients to your cells, lowering your risk of disease.

EZ water can also be made through grounding. As you learned in Chapter 3, the earth contains lots of electrons and when you place your bare feet on the ground you absorb these electrons through your skin. Dr. Pollack surmises that once these negative electrons enter your body they help form EZ water. This is why it is good to go barefoot, because not only do you capture electrons from the earth, you also create more EZ water in your body.

While Dr. Pollack is working in a lab at the University of Washington, I'm treating patients four miles away in my clinic. Although for years I have been recommending patients drink more water, especially filtered and spring water, a few years ago I read Pollack's research and got very excited. Recently, I began using a commercially prepared form of water that is very similar to EZ water with a few of my patients. After drinking a liter of the water each day for a month, there was a sharp reduction of their symptoms and inflammatory markers on their labs. This was only a small sample, but presently I am helping set up a clinical pilot study to see the effects of this water on inflammation and people's health. While I am not aware of any commercial forms of EZ water being available to buy, Dr. Pollack and other scientists suggest that chilling water to 38 degrees produces more electrons that may help your body to make EZ water. Most importantly though, the simplest way to increase EZ water in your body is: Drink lots of water, mostly spring and let light and earth, do their thing.

Imprinting Water

You now know how to maximize your energy using water, but if you want to make your water even more vital, consider this: There is a theory in medicine and water science called "imprinting" that states that energy (or messages) can be transmitted through water. Many cultures and religions have sought to infuse religious or spiritual messages into water by praying over, singing to or blessing the water. It was believed that if this water was consumed, the message would be transferred to the body for a beneficial effect or cleansing. Whether you believe the spiritual aspect or not, there is also a scientific explanation to it that Dr. Pollack and others have hypothesized. Perhaps one of the most famous experiments that demonstrates imprinting was done by Luc Montagnier, PhD, who won the 2008 Nobel Prize in Physiology or Medicine for his discovery of the human immunodeficiency virus (HIV).

Montagnier showed that if he put HIV DNA in a glass tube, diluted it with water to 10-16 (or 10 quadrillion), it could not be seen with a microscope, but its electromagnetic signal could be picked up. He then set a sealed glass tube of filtered water next to it and put a low-intensity electric current around the two tubes for 18 hours. When he tested the second tube, he found the electromagnetic message from tube one had transferred to the second tube without any physical contact between them. Next, he added to the second test tube a solution (PCR) that makes virus DNA visible under a microscope. After this step, the HIV DNA was observable under a microscope, proving his theory that messages can be transferred or imprinted through water (add "without any physical contact"). How this process happens is still being studied, but it has been repeated successfully several times.

While Montagnier's experiment involved complex DNA and electromagnetic signals, Pollack and others have argued that we can use simpler methods to help transfer messages that can improve our health into water. Even a few pharmaceutical companies are now trying to imprint their drugs into water or other substances in order to improve their effectiveness and make them less toxic. One imprinting researcher, while somewhat controversial, is

Dr. Masaru Emoto who examined water with microscopic photography. He saw that when positive or negative words or messages were written on the bottle, the water inside changed its shape and structure.

What does this mean to you? Treat your water as you would like to be treated or better yet, like the person you would like to become. You are that second test tube. You can take the concepts of Montagnier's research and put them into action by writing messages on your bottles to help improve your life. For example, at home, we write messages of love, hope, health, prosperity, energy, and gratitude on our water bottles.

Your Own Water Journey

Let me give you some suggestions on how to begin your water journey. First and foremost, keep it simple. Start by drinking more water, preferably spring or filtered, and refrigerated to 38 degrees. The exact amount of water depends on the individual, but generally try to drink, in ounces, 2/3 of your body weight. If you weigh 150 pounds, then this would be about 100 ounces of water a day. If you can't drink that much water, then start off by drinking one or two more glasses than your current daily intake. I personally drink about a gallon every day. I fill four water bottles with spring water and put them in the refrigerator the night before. After drinking plenty of water, you can begin to turn the water in your body into energizing EZ water by grounding and getting natural light through your skin and eyes.

To find out where you can collect your own spring water, I recommend you go to www.findaspring.com for a local source. If that is not practical, you can also buy spring water at a store or have it delivered in five-gallon containers. If the cost of drinking only spring water is prohibitive, I suggest adding some to your filtered water to make it last longer. For suggestions on water filters, go to drramaley. com. As a side note, you can also vortex or spin your water which theoretically produces more electrons. Please see my website for more information on how to do this. Finally, imprint your water by writing positive messages, goals and affirmations on your bottles

Back to Lisa: When I saw her about a month later, she said that she loved her new discovery of water. Her shoulder and joint pain had cleared up and her skin looked and felt more vibrant. Her energy also increased and she didn't crave or need as much coffee. She laughingly said that she couldn't bring herself to sing to the local lake, but she did write sayings of prosperity, love, and health on her water bottles, and bought local spring water from a delivery service. She also bought a water filter for home that removed fluoride and other pollutants. She went outside in the natural light often and grounded a couple of times a week. Best of all, she was able to return to her Pilates class which helped alleviate her stress so work became more enjoyable and she was more relaxed with her clients.

SUMMARY

- 99% of the molecules in your body are water, so you are 99% water.

- Water is essential for your DNA and proteins to replicate properly. Without enough water, you will get abnormal gene expression leading to disease and fatigue.

- The average American drinks about three glasses of water a day, yet urinates about 6.5 glasses of liquid a day.

- Much of our drinking water is full of chemicals, fluoride and pollutants. If you drink that water, then the 99% of your molecules become polluted water.

- Exclusion Zone (EZ) water contains just electrons and no protons, so it is full of energy and is distinct from regular water. This is the water that is inside of your cells, making them healthy and vibrant. EZ water also allows your blood to flow more easily in your body.

- Your body makes EZ water when it is exposed to natural light on your skin, in your eyes and when you are barefoot on ground, like grass, dirt or cement.

SOLUTIONS

- Drink lots of water, mostly spring and let light and earth do their thing.

- Make it a goal to drink about 2/3 of your body weight in ounces. If you weigh 150 pounds this would be about 100 ounces. If this is too much, start off with just an extra glass or two a day, as any increase will make a difference.

- When you first wake up, drink about 16 ounces of cool water with the juice of half a lemon to jumpstart your day.

- Filtered water is always better than tap water. Try to get a filter that removes fluoride, since this mineral affects the vitality of the water.

- Spring water is the best, since it already contains some EZ water and is generally free of pollutants.

- Drink water chilled to about 38 degrees.

- Go outside to get natural light and go barefoot.

- You can write messages (imprinting) on your water bottle that deal with spiritual, financial or personal goals such as "prosperity" or "gratitude."

Chapter 7

Movement and Exercise

*"Step with care and great tact and remember
life's a great balancing act."*

~ Dr. Seuss

Angela was sitting in the chair nearly doubled over in pain when I first met her. She couldn't straighten her back. She worked long hours as a CFO for a very large fish company. She had held this current position for the past six years, but recently had spent more time at her desk and in meetings, working up to ten hours a day. She bought herself an ergonomic chair thinking it might help, but she still felt like her body was falling apart. Upon waking, she found it difficult to get out of bed, and her wife commented on how much Angela grunted when she bent over to do normal activities like loading the dishwasher. Even a simple task, such as picking up a piece of paper, was problematic. She worked out at the gym four times a week, jogging on a treadmill for 40 minutes and doing lightweight training, but lately she found this to be a struggle. She also walked the dog in the morning for about ten minutes. She thought that she was in decent shape, but clearly something wasn't right.

I examined the muscles and joints of her back, and they moved fairly well. When I palpated the muscles in her hips and pelvis, they were like steel and she jumped and flinched in pain. I asked her how many hours she sat every day and how often she got up out of her chair. She replied that she was glued to her chair all day, sitting for two to three hours at a time before she would stand up to get a cup of coffee or go to the bathroom. I asked her if she smoked and she emphatically said no because she knew how bad it was for her health. I told her she might as well be smoking a pack of cigarettes a day unless she got herself out of that chair. As you may have heard, sitting is the new smoking. Dr. James Levine, from the Mayo Clinic, coined this term.

Movement Is Life

Outside of exercising, how much time do you spend standing or moving? With the exception of walking to the car or bus, most people move very little. I often have patients recall their daily activities and they are usually surprised how little they actually move their bodies. Studies show that in the US, 86% of all full-time office workers sit for almost the entire day and then do the same at home, watching TV, gaming, eating, reading, or continuing to use their computer. Comparatively, our ancestors likely kept moving and weren't sedentary. Even our grandparents' generation moved a lot more than we do today. I recently met a 95-year-old woman who has perfect posture, moves well and is mentally sharp. I asked her what she did for exercise and she said, "Honey, I don't exercise, I just don't sit down."

So, what are your health risks for sitting too much and what can you do about them?

A recent study by Kaiser Permanente found that workers who did intense exercise but had sedentary jobs had a higher risk of dying earlier than those who didn't exercise but had jobs in which they moved a lot during the day. Another study in 2010 found that sitting for 11 or more hours a day created a 40% increased mortality risk. In addition to the lowered risks of disease, standing will improve your posture. As in the case of Angela, sitting all day tightens up the hip flexors and bends you forward. I can usually tell if people sit a lot because even at a young age they have a hunched-over posture. This will only worsen with age and with more sitting.

"Get Up Offa That Thing...."

Perhaps one of the biggest proponents for movement is Dr. Joan Vermikos, former director of NASA's Life Sciences Division who studied the health of astronauts in space. In her book Sitting Kills, Moving Heals, she says that it is not just how many hours a day we stand or sit, but how many times we change our position in a day. She suggests that we get up at least 35 times throughout the workday. Our bodies are not designed to be doing the same static activity or to sit or stand in the same position all the time. She proposes that we do more getting up and down motions so the brain and body think that we are defying gravity, thereby making our muscles work harder (and burn more fat). She showed in an experiment that standing up once every hour during the day was the equivalent in cardiovascular and metabolic changes to 15 minutes of treadmill walking. Other researchers have expanded on this idea and call it Non-Exercise Activity Thermogenesis (NEAT). These are activities such as bending over to pick up a piece of paper off the floor, reaching for a plate, brushing your teeth, walking to your car, getting out of your chair, going up stairs, etc. When patients tell me that they don't have time to go to the gym, I tell them that they are surrounded by one.

If you have an office job and sit most of the day, I highly suggest a sit-stand desk. These are lifesavers for your back, and you will have less pain at the end of the day. When you sit, set a timer and get up every 20 minutes and stand, walk to the water cooler, or do deep knee bends for 15 seconds. Other suggestions include always taking the stairs, walking over to talk with a colleague instead of texting or emailing, and taking a less direct route to go to the restroom. Find avenues of increasing movement in small ways. At home, while working on the computer or watching TV, stand up during commercials and walk in place. I like to go up and down the stairs, play tag with my kids, or head outside to walk a few blocks. You can be as creative as you like. Overall, this will help strengthen your core muscles, stretch your back, and work your arms and legs. If you become a NEAT freak, you can get the equivalent of an hour's worth of walking on a treadmill without even leaving the office or your home.

High Intensity Work Out

If you want to burn more calories and increase your energy beyond NEAT, research has shown that the best form of exercise is High-Intensity Interval Training (HIIT). While this form of exercise has been very effective for my patients, I always recommend you check with your healthcare provider before beginning any new exercise regimen. HIIT involves short bursts of rigorous exercise. The routine starts with a five-minute warm-up, then moves on to a strenuous physical activity for 30 seconds to a minute, pushing as hard as you can. Next, rest for 30 seconds to a minute. Repeat this five more times. You can do this on a recumbent bike, on an elliptical machine in your gym, or by walking quickly or running up a steep neighborhood hill. When I say as hard as you can, I mean as hard as you can. You only get the benefit of HIIT if you really push yourself. The advantage of HIIT is that even though it is a very short workout, you keep burning calories for another 24 to 48 hours after you finish.

A 15-minute workout with HIIT burns only about 100 calories during the workout, but overall you end up burning 400-500 calories over a longer period of time. Compare this to a regular work out. Let's say you get on a treadmill or elliptical machine and do a moderate routine for 45 minutes. You burn roughly 200 calories, but when you are done you cease to burn extra calories. I love doing HIIT because it is a more efficient use of my time, burns more calories, and I feel stronger and more flexible. Of course, this is only part of my overall activities. I spend less time exercising and more time "recreating." I like to think of HIIT as "exercise" and other activities as "recreation", which are still movement and healthy, but not as intense. For example, tennis, dancing, walking, jogging, or yoga can be done at an enjoyable level without having to focus on making it "exercise." Make your movement fun and you are more likely to do it.

This is how HIIT exercise works its magic. We have different types of muscle fibers called Type I and Type II. Type I are called "slow twitch" and are used for standing, jogging, or walking. Our ancestors likely used these to track an animal or forage for food. Type II are "fast twitch" and allow us to exert lots of strength in a short amount of time. For example, our ancestors likely used Type II to protect themselves from a wild tiger or to swim across a fast-moving river. Type I fibers use very little energy (calories), whereas Type II fibers use a lot of energy (more calories). Your body will preferentially use Type I fibers first, and as the exercise and intensity continues, it switches to Type II. Now that we live in the land of plenty and don't fight off animals, we rarely use these Type II fibers. Jogging or other low intensity exercises only use Type I fibers. The only real way to access Type II fibers is to exercise at an intensity that will fatigue your Type I fibers, causing your body to switch to the Type II. This whole process can roughly take place in just 30 - 60 seconds.

Here is the other cool thing about Type II fibers. When we use them, they push a lot of fuel called pyruvate into our mitochondria to produce ATP and electrons. The mitochondria can only take in so much pyruvate at one time, so it sends this fuel to the liver to be stored. Once the HIIT is done and your body has calmed down, your liver keeps releasing the pyruvate for one to two days longer. Essentially your body still thinks that you are exercising even though you are not, so it produces more electrons and burns more calories. This is how you end up burning that extra 400-500 calories with HIIT.

Now, not everybody can run and do interval work because of certain health conditions or pain. However, most people can ride a stationary bike and do HIIT by pedaling as fast as possible for 30 - 60 seconds. If you search for "HIIT exercises" on YouTube, you will find many examples you can easily do at home. When you first start doing HIIT, I suggest you start with less exertion and build up so you do not hurt yourself. While HIIT once a week is enough, it's OK to do it twice a week with three days in between for recovery. If you have any serious health conditions, speak to your healthcare practitioner first to make sure that this type of exercise is okay.

So what happened to Angela? She told me she got a sit-stand desk and changed positions all day long and, if she could help it, never sat for more than 20 minutes. She started doing a few deep knee bends and toe touches in her office and would often take the stairs. In the summer she mowed the lawn, which she hadn't done since her pain began. She now felt better and had the energy to enjoy working in her yard. She slowly started doing the HIIT routine and worked up to six intervals on her stationary bike at home. She still went to the gym but not nearly as much, freeing her up to spend more time being active with her friends. She lost weight and felt better. The last time I saw her, she told me, "Movement rules, sitting sucks." Maybe not Shakespeare but you get the point.

SUMMARY

- 86% of full-time office workers in the US sit almost the entire day.

- Sitting is the new smoking.

- According to a study, sitting for 11 or more hours a day created a 40% increased mortality risk.

- Workers who did intense exercise but had sedentary jobs had a higher risk of dying earlier than those who didn't exercise but didn't have sedentary jobs.

- Standing up once every hour during the day is the equivalent in cardiovascular and metabolic changes to 15 minutes of treadmill walking.

- High-Intensity Interval Training (HIIT) burns more calories over time compared to a longer but less stressful workout like jogging on a treadmill.

- Type I muscle fibers are slow twitch and used more for low-intensity exercise and less strenuous activities. Type II fibers are fast twitch and are triggered by strenuous exercise or HIIT

SOLUTIONS

- Move, move, and move.

- Get a sit/stand desk for your work or home.

- Use Non-Exercise Activity Thermogenesis (NEAT) like picking up paper off the floor, taking the stairs, doing deep knee bends, and getting out of your chair several times repeatedly.

- Try to get up out of your chair at least every 20 minutes and do some type of movement for 15 - 30-seconds.

- Use HIIT exercise once or twice a week to lose more weight in less time.

- Park your car further away than you are used to.

Chapter 8

Electromagnetic Fields

*"There is no question EMFs have a major effect on
neurological functioning. They slow our brainwaves and
affect our long- term mental clarity. We should minimize
exposures as much as possible to optimize neurotransmitter
levels and prevent deterioration of health."*

~ Dr. Eric Braverman, The Edge Effect

Raj was living in a condo and had been there for 11 years
without many health issues. He was a successful entrepre-
neur and worked in the technology sector. However, in the
last four years he developed a severe sleeping problem. He
would wake up almost every hour and he felt like this was
making him crazy. His libido had dropped off and he was
having trouble getting an erection. He would get headaches
and had low-grade nausea. He used to cycle long distances
on the weekend, but gave that up because of the fatigue he

experienced. He had seen a neurologist, gastroenterologist, internist, and psychiatrist, and had lots of lab work done as well as two MRIs. He had tried numerous medications but none of them helped. No one had been able to identify why he was having these problems. I could see the frustration on Raj's face and he looked like he wanted to just lie down on the exam table and fall asleep. He said his wife and friends had noticed a big change in him and they were very worried. His blood pressure was extremely high, his pulse was fast, and he had developed ringing in his ears. Raj, like so many other people I have seen in the last decade, was exposing his brain and body to Electromagnetic Fields (EMFs) 24 hours a day, seven days a week. It was taking a toll on his health. Here is what Raj's typical day looked like.

In the morning, he would walk to work with his phone in his pocket and a device on his wrist. He was excited when the first wireless fitness tracker came out, and he wore it all day and night since he wanted to keep a good record of his health statistics. When the smart watch became widely available, he bought one and wore it 24 hours a day. He spent most of the day sitting at his desk in front of a computer. He would spend anywhere from 60 to 90 minutes a day on his cell phone, talking with clients. At home, he slept with his cell phone next to him and his Wi-Fi router was on day and night. In the evenings, he used his laptop for entertainment. He also enjoyed gaming for a couple of hours. Recently he had purchased a voice-activated system for his living room that he could give commands to. This was left on day and night as well.

Does Raj's life sound anything like yours? Raj was connected 24/7. The wireless devices were amazing and created efficiency, but it was evident that they were affecting his nervous system and health.

Wireless and Tired

How many wireless devices do you own? Most people likely have at least three but often many more. These wireless devices communicate with an ever-expanding number of cell towers that you have probably seen in your neighborhood. These devices and cell towers emit what are called electromagnetic fields (EMFs) or electromagnetic radiation. There are different types of EMFs. Some come naturally from the earth and atmosphere. These have existed longer than humankind. Another type of EMF is created by humans and started with the invention of electricity. Then about 70 years ago, microwave communications were created. In the last 20 years, there has been an exponential growth of EMFs, and they are more ubiquitous now in the form of cell phones, cell towers and wireless routers. These forms of EMFs are particularly harmful to your body, and this is evident in numerous patients I have treated.

As I mentioned above, cell phones and most wireless devices emit EMFs. There is an active debate about the harmful effects they produce. The debate tends to center around whether or not talking on a cell phone causes cancer. So far, there is not enough evidence to definitively prove that cell phone use alone will cause cancer. However, the World Health Organization (WHO) states that cell phones are classified as a Group 2B carcinogen, meaning that there is a correlation between cell phone use and cancer. Perhaps a better question to ask is: What happens when you have your cell phone on you all day + you are in front of a computer for many hours + you wear wireless devices? The cumulative effect of this level of exposure has not been thoroughly studied. In my clinic, I see many patients coming in for fatigue and sleep issues that appear to be directly related to excessive EMF exposure. New studies are currently showing that EMF frequencies are having an adverse effect on our health.

One of the reasons why cell phones may be harmful to you is that the wavelength produced by a cell phone is very different than the wavelengths of the human brain. Two recent studies demonstrated that when the brain is exposed to a cell phone, the alpha waves, important for focus and delta waves, important for sleep, were altered, which resulted in lack of concentration and insomnia for almost all of the participants.

In addition, the American Academy of Environmental Medicine states that exposure to EMFs creates a sort of "leaking" of the barrier (blood brain barrier) around the brain that protects it from toxins, bacteria, and viruses. When this leakage happens, it can damage your brain and lead to headaches, dizziness, sleep issues, poor memory, and more serious health problems like dementia. There is also the thermal or heat effect of the cell phone when placed next to your ear. It is known to heat up the tissue of your brain within several minutes, creating hormonal imbalances. Our ancestors did not have these kinds of EMF stressors, and rapid development of technology has not given our bodies enough time to adequately evolve to meet these challenges.

Another interesting patient story is that of Yin. She was an executive secretary who was experiencing numbness and tingling and a lot of pain and weakness in her wrists. She had to stop working because she could no longer type on a keyboard. Her doctors told her that she needed carpal tunnel surgery on both wrists. When she came to see me she had upcoming wrist surgeries scheduled. Upon examination, I noticed that she had a wireless activity tracker on her left wrist. When I orthopedically tested the strength of her fingers and wrists there was a weakness in almost all of her muscles. Then, taking a reflex hammer and tapping her wrists (a common neurological test), her symptoms of numbness and tingling were aggravated, which indicated carpal tunnel problems. I then had her remove the wireless wrist device, waited about one minute and retested her. She no longer had any weakness in her hands and when I tapped her wrists with a reflex hammer she no longer had the numbness or tingling sensations. She could move her hands and fingers and reported about 50% less pain. She was extremely surprised. Next, I had her put the device back on her wrist, and we waited about five minutes. Retesting her, she had the same weakness and pain in her hands and when I tapped her wrists with a hammer she once again felt the numbness. I told her this probably indicated that her real problem was exposure to the EMFs emitted by the wrist device and not a true carpal tunnel problem. I explained to her the neurology and how the syncing of her device to her phone triggers inflammatory pathways. My detailed explanation wasn't necessary, as she had already decided to stop using her fitness tracker for the time being. Feeling better, she cancelled her surgeries and returned back to work.

I am not suggesting that you get rid of all of your wireless devices. I am recommending you use them more wisely and efficiently. I use my smart phone and love it. My clinic runs much more smoothly with Wi-Fi, and my house is connected as well. There are ways to use these devices while lessening their negative impact on your health by taking certain precautions and changing some of your habits. Let me make some suggestions using Raj as an example.

Reconfiguring Your Wireless Life

Now, when Raj is at work or needs to have his cell phone on, he keeps it at least four feet from his body and uses the speakerphone when possible. He also uses ear buds that have air tubes the last few inches before the earpiece that dramatically cut down on the EMFs to the brain. He stopped putting the cell phone up to his ear and never uses a blue tooth earpiece because it sits too close to the brain and emits a very strong electromagnetic field. Texting is the best option for communication, so he texts instead of calls whenever possible. He keeps his phone on Airplane Mode when he doesn't need immediate communication. Airplane Mode completely stops all EMF emissions. At night when he goes to bed, he puts his cell phone on Airplane Mode or places it at least five feet from his body. He no longer wears his smart watch on his wrist, because he realizes that it is like wearing a cell phone on his body, creating a constant strong and searching EMF signal. I explained to Raj that it is fine to use a fitness tracker to monitor sleep habits, heart rate, and steps at times, as sometimes this data can be very valuable. However, I told him to turn off continuous syncing and only sync the data with his phone or computer once a day.

After making these adjustments, Raj immediately began to feel better. Within a few days, his nausea got better, and his sleep and libido improved. He was feeling more energetic and was surprised that the simple changes he had made in his daily habits were not much of a hassle. He was motivated, so he asked what else he could do to improve his health. I suggested that when he didn't need to be online, he use the "turn Wi-Fi off" option on the menu bar of his computer, which would lower his EMF exposure. At night, I had him turn off his voice-activated device, gaming console, and router so he wouldn't be exposed to EMFs while sleeping. The last thing I told him was to keep his cell phone as far away from him as possible when it is searching or ringing another phone or when it is low in bars or reception. During these times, the phone emits the highest amount of EMFs. Then, you guessed it, I told him to go outside. He did this and he told me that he felt much younger and was excited to be back cycling on the weekends.

SUMMARY

- Americans spend, on average, almost three hours a day on wireless devices like cell phones and tablets.

- Electromagnetic Fields (EMFs) emit wavelengths that are much different than your brain's wavelengths, so they alter how your brain functions and lead to insomnia and poor concentration.

- EMFs are emitted from wireless devices, especially cellphones, and can negatively affect your health. According to the World Health Organization, cell phones are classified as a Group 2B carcinogen.

- EMFs can cause a leaking of the barrier around the brain that protects it from toxins and bacteria. This in turn can cause neurological problems like headaches, insomnia, dizziness, and more serious health issues like Alzheimer's and dementia.

- Cell phones emit the strongest EMF radiation when there is poor reception (few bars), you are first making a call, or the phone is searching for a signal.

- Texting emits the least amount of radiation.

SOLUTIONS

- You can reduce your EMF exposure by keeping your cell phone at least two to five inches away from your ear when talking. You can do this by turning on speakerphone, or by using ear buds that have an air tube the last few inches near the earpiece. Go to my website for sources.

- Text instead of talking on your phone when possible.

- Use the Airplane Mode on your phone when you don't need to talk or text because this eliminates all forms of EMF. You can turn the Airplane Mode on and off quickly to periodically check for recent texts, emails, or messages.

- When the phone is in "calling" mode, keep it as far away as possible until the other person has answered.

- Turn off your Wi-Fi devices at night to lessen your exposure.

- If you use a fitness tracker, turn off the sync mode on your phone so the wrist device isn't continuously communicating with it. Sync it up at the end of the day to gather your data.

Chapter 9

Stress and Hormones

"It's not stress that kills us, it is our reaction to it."

~ Hans Selye

A number of years ago, my wife and I lived in Juneau, AK. In early spring that year, we were inspired to take a week-long kayak journey through Glacier Bay. It is a remote area with no connection to the outside world and, at that time of year, no powered boats or ships were allowed in the bay. During our trip we did not see a single person, plane, or boat. We were literally on our own. Already in a precarious position, we quickly learned the true meaning of stress and how it serves us as humans. On the third day out, we decided to take a two-mile hike up to an ice cave. Entering the dark cave, we both slipped and landed in a deep pool of freezing cold water surrounded by a wall of ice. We started to panic and weren't sure how we were going to make it out. We treaded water for a few seconds and luckily found a shallow area in which we could stand on our tip-toes. With some ingenuity and a huge adrenaline surge, we were able to pull ourselves out of the water. Once out of the water, I could still feel the adrenaline rushing through my body and my heart pumping. What surprised me though, was that within a few minutes I was relaxed again and the adrenaline had dissipated. My recovery seemed so different than other stressful events I had experienced at work or in my daily routine. This all made sense to me years later when I studied physiology.

Your body is designed to handle stress, but perhaps stress that is more like the physical stress our ancestors experienced. Falling into ice water or being chased by a wild animal requires a tremendous surge of physical exertion and a quick response, after which your body returns to its normal state. In contrast, a mentally induced modern world type of stress might include receiving a confrontational phone call from a client, being stuck in traffic late for an important meeting, or having an abnormal mammogram. The threat that involves a physical response, like running from an animal, quickly burns up the adrenaline in your body, whereas sitting and feeling stressed out in traffic does not allow for any physical exertion to properly eliminate adrenaline. Our release valve remains closed, adding to our stress and allowing adrenaline to remain in the body for too long.

Hans Selye, a famous endocrinologist who wrote the widely read The Stress of Life in 1956, further hypothesized that stress can basically be categorized into acute and chronic. Acute stressors are examples we used above, where the event was short-lived and brought on either a physical or mental response. Chronic stressors are more long term and can be experienced in many ways. Examples are: living with cancer; caring for a sick parent; or an accumulation of daily physical and mental stresses that build up over time.

Your Hormones and Stress

Selye explained that there are three primary glands that deal with stress called the hypothalamus and pituitary, located in the brain, and the adrenal glands near the kidneys. These three make up the hypothalamic-pituitary-adrenal axis (HPA axis) and they communicate closely with each other.

Your hypothalamus receives information from the nervous system regarding your perception of a stress or threat, and then communicates the information to the pituitary. The pituitary then tells the adrenal glands to secrete hormones to deal with the stress. The most important adrenal hormones are adrenaline and cortisol. When secreted in larger amounts, these hormones, especially cortisol, cause your blood to move from the digestive system to your muscles, raise your blood pressure, increase your heart rate, dilate your eyes, and turn the food you eat into fat. This is what Selye called the "alarm state," and this response helps you stay alive.

However, if the hormones stay elevated for several weeks, months, or years, you may develop insomnia, elevated blood pressure, irritability, or headaches. Prolonged elevated cortisol levels also affect the mitochondria and cause them to produce fewer electrons. If these hormones stay heightened indefinitely, the adrenals become fatigued and hormone production declines. This is the last phase of adrenal imbalance that Selye called the "exhaustive state." It is exactly as it sounds: You are completely burned out. You lose your motivation, your libido decreases, your thinking becomes cloudy, muscle and joint pain can plague you, and you just don't feel well. When in this state, you have probably been to several doctors and no one can find anything medically wrong. What has occurred is that due to prolonged stress, your hypothalamus, pituitary, and adrenal glands no longer communicate with each other, and your stress response hormones have hit rock bottom. Your whole body is out of rhythm. This is adrenal burnout, and it is one of the more common diagnoses I make with my patient population.

If you suffer from menopausal symptoms, proper adrenal function is also important because as the ovaries age and produce less estrogen, the adrenal glands pick up the slack and help supplement this hormone, making the transition through this stage of life easier. If your adrenals are fatigued, you don't have this back-up system and probably don't feel well.

The Thyroid-Adrenal Connection

To add fuel to the fire, the excess or lack of the hormone cortisol can affect the thyroid gland. This gland helps produce lots of energy in your body and assists in metabolism. The thyroid, like the adrenal glands, receives information from the hypothalamus and pituitary via a hormone called Thyroid Stimulating Hormone (TSH). The TSH signals to the thyroid to secrete thyroid hormone T4, which then gets converted to the active form of thyroid hormone called T3. If cortisol is too high or too low, it can cause the following: It can block TSH from being secreted from the pituitary; it can block T4 to T3 conversion; or it can prevent T3 from getting into the cells of the body. Any one of these scenarios will create fatigue and malaise and may look like hypothyroidism, but in reality, it is adrenal fatigue and stress that cause the thyroid to shut down in the first place. Of course, it is possible to have a true hypothyroid problem, but it is often over-diagnosed. To get to the root of most hypothyroid problems, adrenal fatigue needs to be addressed.

To restore the health of your adrenal and thyroid glands, light and earth are essential. Recall in Chapter 2 that blue light from computer screens, cell phones, etc. shines directly into your eyes, causing inflammation and cortisol imbalances. The more you block out blue light and allow natural light into your eyes, the quicker these glands will heal. Within weeks of patients' implementing this lifestyle change, I have seen their abnormal adrenal and thyroid lab values improve and their energy and sleep problems diminish. The next step is grounding, which I discussed in Chapter 3. Remember that negative electrons from the earth will flow through your bare feet into your body, creating a calming effect on the adrenal glands. Just a few minutes a day will make a big change in your adrenal and thyroid function.

It is also important to limit your caffeine consumption, as this can abnormally raise your cortisol levels. Excessive sugar intake raises your blood glucose levels, also causing an increase in cortisol. While I do not recommend any specific dietary plans, remember in Chapter 6 that fat creates lots of energy in the body and it also improves blood sugar levels, which in turn, balance cortisol levels. If you are interested, there is a book called Fat as Fuel by Dr. Joseph Mercola that gives some excellent information on this.

Breathing With ROY G. BIV

I would like to offer one quick tip that takes only five minutes and can fit into your busy schedule. It almost instantly lowers your stress level and helps you think more clearly. Start off by sitting in a comfortable chair or lying down. You can do this in your office or even in your parked car. Now, visualize the colors of the rainbow (also called chakra colors) in this order: red, orange, yellow, green, blue, indigo, and violet. The mnemonic is ROY G. BIV. First, take a slow deep breath in through your nose and visualize the color red coming up through your feet, all the way to the top of your head. Hold your breath for a few seconds, and then breathe out slowly through your mouth all the way. See the red flow out through your feet again. Now do the same thing, but this time with orange, and continue until you have gone through all of the ROY G. BIV colors. There are many other de-stressing activities that you may already be doing, such as yoga, tai chi, qi gong and meditation. Find what works for you and your body and try to do it daily.

There are also unique herbs, vitamins, and minerals that can support the adrenal and thyroid glands. For the adrenals, my favorite herbs are Ashwagandha and Rhodiola. These are adaptogens meaning that if cortisol is too high they will bring it down, or if too low they will raise cortisol. My favorite vitamins that also balance the adrenals are B5 and B6. They bring the adrenals to a healthier state and will give you an immediate boost in energy. For B5, take 500 mg, and for B6 take 100mg one time, twice per day. For the thyroid, iodine balances the gland very well, and I recommend a very safe dose of 200 mcg a day for those who need it. You can also try eating some arame seaweed, which is high in iodine.

If our adrenal glands really do interpret stress more like a physical threat, then the best way to balance our adrenals is to do High-Intensity Interval Training (HIIT), discussed in Chapter 7. Remember, this is just one to two times per week for about 15 minutes and can be done in a gym or at home. Also, moving during the day at work will help with the immediate stress you may feel after a not-so-friendly phone call or while facing a looming project deadline. I guarantee you will be so much happier if you implement these suggestions in your life. Patients have often told me others comment on their vitality after they follow these suggestions. Give them a try!

All of these remedies help you release the stress from your body and mind. That is the ticket to getting more energy and preventing disease.

SUMMARY

- Your primary glands that help you deal with stress are called your adrenal glands. They secrete cortisol and adrenaline to help you respond to stress.

- For short periods of time, cortisol and adrenaline can help your body resist stress. If they stay elevated for too long though, you can start to develop health problems like elevated blood pressure, headaches, low libido, migraines, and eventually, fatigue and joint pain.

- As the ovaries age and produce less estrogen, the adrenals take over this role, helping with menopausal symptoms.

- Imbalances in cortisol can hamper the function of your thyroid, making you more tired. Many cases of hypothyroid are actually a problem with the adrenal glands.

SOLUTIONS

- Breathe deeply using the Rainbow meditation exercise. Visualize the colors of the rainbow: red, orange, yellow, green, blue, indigo, and violet (ROY G. BIV), and take a slow deep breath in through your nose and visualize the color red coming up through your feet, all the way to the top of your head. Hold your breath for a few seconds, and then breathe out slowly though your mouth all the way and see the red flow out through your feet again. Now do the same thing, but this time with orange, and continue until you have gone through all of the colors.

- Do yoga, qi gong, tai chi, or meditate.

- Decrease caffeine intake to just one or two cups a day.

- Block out blue light from computer screens.

- Go outside.

- Exercise using HIIT to help release excessive cortisol and adrenaline from your body.

- Take adrenal support like Ashwagandha and Rhodiola and vitamins B5 and B6.

Chapter 10
Vitamins and Minerals

*"Provided one has the correct level of vitamin, mineral and
nutritional input, the body can overcome disease"*

~ Linus Pauling

Keesha is a 61-year-old architect who has her own successful business. She has three children and four grandchildren whom she loves dearly. When she first came in for treatment, she was experiencing a wide range of health problems. Just like many of the patients I have previously discussed, Keesha had a lot of stress and was spending a great deal of time in front of her computer. Not only was she tired and losing her focus at work, she was also experiencing what felt like panic attacks. As a result, she was prescribed an anti-anxiety medication, but it made her constipated and gain weight. She was finding that she didn't have the energy to play with her grandchildren or to work out on her elliptical machine. She also began to feel her heart flutter during the day and especially at night. She was prescribed a beta-blocker medication, and while it did help with the heart flutter, she became even more tired. She would wake up many times during the night and was scheduled for a sleep study. She was recently diagnosed with osteoporosis and was prescribed another medication. She didn't like the fact that she was taking three drugs and wondered how many more she would be taking in the years to come. She was using supplements but wasn't sure what to take or how they might be of benefit. A blood test revealed that her vitamin D was low at 22 ng/ml and her magnesium RBC (red blood cell) was also low at 4.2 mg/dL.

While it would have been easy to start prescribing different supplements or pharmaceuticals for each condition that she had, I took a step back to see the big picture of what was happening to Keesha. Her lifestyle was depleting her of electrons and aggravating her symptoms. She needed to start with the fundamentals. The first things I had her do were focus on being in sunlight, drinking healthy water, grounding outside, and changing her diet, as well as increasing her exercise regimen. Although that was a good start for her and she began to feel better, she still needed to jumpstart her body. This is where specific supplementation would boost her energy and electron production.

In this chapter, I will talk about the basic vitamins and supplements that are helpful for you to increase your energy and feel significantly better. My suggestions are clearly neither exhaustive nor intended to address every health issue you may have, but I want to keep them accessible and give you a simple foundation for increasing your electron production. While each vitamin and mineral is unique, they have two things in common: They all help produce energy in the body and they are deficient in the US diet. According to the NHANES 2001-2008 nutritional study funded by the Centers for Disease Control, 40% to 90% of the US population is deficient or below the RDA for vitamins A, D, K2 and magnesium. This does not refer to optimal amounts, or what is best for optimal health, but the minimal amount in order to avoid outright pathology and disease. Without these essential vitamins and minerals, your body can't function properly. While it is best to get them from food, there are taste preferences, cultural and religious norms, and food availability issues that can make obtaining them a challenge. I will offer suggestions on how to find these nutrients in a pill or powder form.

Vitamin D

The most important vitamin of all is D. I can't possibly cover all the functions of vitamin D in the body, but suffice it to say that without it, energy production goes down significantly and healthy gene expression declines. Vitamin D helps the mitochondria produce more energy, strengthens bones, and helps regulate your immune system. Vitamin D deficiency in the US is rampant, with almost 3/4 of the population falling below the normal range. Without enough vitamin D, you are prone to cancer, diabetes, fatigue, and osteoporosis. I think it is imperative that everyone get their vitamin D levels tested, and while debatable, I believe the optimal level should be somewhere between 30-70 ng/ml. Some experts think it should be higher, but I am not convinced of this yet. If you take the correct amounts of the vitamins that work synergistically with vitamin D that I discuss in this chapter, then you will need less vitamin D. Foods high in vitamin D include fatty fish, especially salmon, halibut, oysters and sardines. Grass-fed dairy products are a good source as well as egg yolks and liver. During the winter, I suggest about 5,000 IU a day and in the summer about 1,000 IU. The absolute best source is the sun. As discussed in Chapter 2, when sunlight hits your bare skin (without sunscreen), there is a high amount of vitamin D made in your body within minutes.

Magnesium

Of next importance is magnesium. This mineral is the foundation for energy production in your body and is essential for making ATP in the mitochondria. It has a very relaxing effect on muscles, so it helps immensely with elevated blood pressure, irregular heartbeat, muscle cramps, restless leg syndrome, eye twitches, and constipation. Magnesium is needed to balance out calcium in your body, and without it, the calcium levels become too high. Magnesium is also needed to activate vitamin D, and without it, vitamin D can remain low in the body. Magnesium has been depleted from our soil, and 60 percent of the US population consumes less than the RDA. It is used up quickly in the body if we are under stress or take certain medications like antibiotics, anti-depressants, and anti-anxiety medications. I use magnesium all the time in our clinic and see dramatic changes in blood pressure, tight muscles, and heart conditions.

I suggest getting a blood test for your magnesium levels, but you must ask for a "Magnesium RBC" and not just a magnesium serum test. The magnesium RBC measures what is actually inside of the cell, so it is more accurate. The optimal range should be above 6.5 mg/dl. Foods high in magnesium are spinach, kale, avocado, seaweed, and black beans. For certain, this is the one mineral I recommend. Take about 300 mg twice a day of any form of magnesium, preferably citrate or glycinate. Many of these come in powdered forms, making it easier to ingest. It is very difficult to overdose on magnesium, but the first sign of too much is loose stools, so it is obvious if you have over-consumed it.

Vitamin A

The next nutrient I recommend is vitamin A. It is also deficient in the typical American diet, with almost half the population not meeting the RDA requirements. One of the most important functions of this vitamin is its high concentration in the retina of the eye, needed for vision, but also for the receptors in the eye that have to do with our circadian rhythm. A deficiency of vitamin A can lead to insomnia and some autoimmune diseases. Vitamin A works directly with vitamin D and, like magnesium, makes vitamin D more active. It also plays a key role in helping thyroid hormone enter the cell so it can be utilized.

There are some plant sources, like carrots, that contain beta-carotene, which can be converted to vitamin A. While carrots may certainly help you meet some of your vitamin A requirements, they can also fall short because many people poorly convert beta-carotene to vitamin A.

Pure vitamin A is only found in animal sources. The most abundant form is in the liver of almost all animals, but also found in cod liver oil, grass-fed dairy products, and egg yolks. If none of these foods sound appealing, then take liver capsules or vitamin A made from fish oil. Don't confuse buying straight fish oil with buying vitamin A. The label will specifically say vitamin A made from fish oil. Take approximately 3,000 IU a day.

Vitamin K2

The most underrepresented vitamin that many people haven't heard about is vitamin K2. You may be familiar with the vitamin K1 because they give this to babies when they're born, but don't confuse K2 with K1. K2 activates vitamin D making it available to the body which allows the vitamin D to enter cells to benefit your health. Vitamin K2 also turns calcium into its activated form, sending it to the correct cells. If calcium is left in the inactivated form, it creates plaquing of the arteries and arthritis in the joints. K2 is mostly found in fermented foods and grass-fed liver, cheeses, butter, and egg yolks. The main constituents of K2 that have a therapeutic effect are MK-4 and MK-7. I recommend taking approximately 1,000 mcg of MK-4 and 100 mcg of MK-7. These can be difficult to find. If need be, go to the resource section of drramaley.com for current vendors.

Getting back to Keesha: She was happy to drink more water and get more light and she saw some improvement but she still wasn't feeling great. She was one of those people that needed to jumpstart her body, so I had her increase her intake of wild-caught, fatty fish and take vitamins D, A and K2 as well as magnesium. Within three weeks her lab values greatly improved, her vitamin D increased to 50 ng/dl, and her magnesium RBC to 6.2. More importantly, her heart rate normalized, she slept through the night, she wasn't as anxious, and she went off the beta-blockers without having a return of her heart flutter. Eventually she weaned herself off her two other medications. Keesha is a perfect example of how important the right nutrition and supplementation of vitamins and minerals can be to improve your health. She began to feel better and have more energy, could exercise, be on target at work and play with her grandkids.

SUMMARY

- The main vitamins and minerals needed to help produce energy in our bodies are A, D, K2, and magnesium. They work synergistically to make more electrons.

- A recent study sponsored by the Centers for Disease Control stated that 40% to 90% of the US population is deficient or below the RDA for vitamins A, D, K2, and magnesium.

- Vitamin D is crucial to maintaining healthy gene expression and making your mitochondria function optimally.

- Vitamin A helps turn on vitamin D and allows thyroid hormone to get into your cells. It is needed for healthy eyes and a normal circadian rhythm.

- Magnesium is extremely important as it helps relax your muscles, makes your heart beat normally, and, most of all, makes your mitochondria produce more energy.

- Vitamin K2 is needed to activate vitamin D in your body. It also makes sure that calcium is activated and that it doesn't end up creating problems in your arteries.

SOLUTIONS

- Take 5,000 IU of vitamin D in the winter and 1,000 in the summer. The best food sources are egg yolks, cod liver oil, grass-fed dairy products and fish. Of course the best source of vitamin D is the sun.

- Magnesium deficiency is quite common, so you want to take at least 300 mg twice a day in the form of magnesium glycinate or citrate. Foods high in magnesium are spinach, kale and avocado.

- You can take up to 3,000 mg a day of vitamin A made from fish oil. It is important that you get vitamin A not just from beta-carotene, as some people can't convert it to vitamin A.

- For vitamin K2, take about 1,000 mcg of MK-4 and 100 mcg of MK-7 on a daily basis to help activate vitamin D and calcium.

Chapter 11

Conclusion

"You have to participate relentlessly in the manifestations
of your own blessings."

~ Elizabeth Gilbert

"Whatever you can do, or dream you can... begin it.
Boldness has genius, power, and magic in it."

~ Goethe

If you are trying to obtain more energy in your life, I suggest you pick one thing from any of the Solutions sections or Takeaways below, and implement it today. Add something else tomorrow. Pick and choose what works for you, as everyone is different. Remain positive and notice how your energy increases incrementally. I know the solutions work because I see my patients' and my own health improve. Everything I suggest that you do in this book I do myself. It may be challenging at times, but there are patch-es of grass and beams of light to be found even during a busy day or living in a city. There are always ways to recon-nect to nature's rhythm. Start where you are. Here are the takeaways from each chapter:

Dr. Ramaley's Ten Ways to Reconnect with Nature

1. Go outside.

2. Take in natural light and reduce blue light exposure.

3. Go barefoot on grass, dirt or the sidewalk.

4. Eat a rainbow of robust foods.

5. Consume a healthy ratio of omega-6 to omega-3 fats. Fat is your friend, not your foe.

6. Drink cold spring water.

7. Make movement part of your day.

8. Reduce exposure to EMFs by turning off your cell phone and wireless devices when possible.

9. Take time to de-stress with yoga, meditation or my Rainbow Exercise.

10. Get adequate amounts of Vitamin D, Magnesium, Vitamin A and K2.

As I said at the beginning, this book is a roadmap, a guide to regain amazing energy. You may have questions or want to learn more about how to implement these changes in your life. You may also want more information or have some health challenges that cannot be fully addressed in this book. Please see a healthcare practitioner or you can contact me at www.drramaley.com for health consulting via phone or Skype.

I hope your journey is full of energy, light and dirt between your toes.

This is not the end, but the beginning.

End Notes

[1] Klepeis NE, Nelson WC, Ott WR, et al. The National Human Activity Pattern Survey (NHAPS): a resource for assessing exposure to environmental pollutants. Journal of Exposure Analysis and Environmental Epidemiology 2001; 11: 231–252.

[2] The Total Audience Report: Q1 2016. The Nielsen Company website. Published June 27 2016.

[3] Mejia R. Green exercise may be good for your head: a new study finds that surprisingly small doses of outdoor activity boost mood, self-esteem. *Environmental Science and Technology.* 2010; 44(10): 3649.

[4] Rivers JK. Is there more than one road to melanoma? *The Lancet.* 2004; 363(9410): 728-30.

[5] Nair R, Maseeh A. "Vitamin D: the "sunshine" vitamin." *Journal of Pharmacology & Pharmacotherapeutics.* 2012;3(2):118-126.

[6] The Feynman Lectures on Physics. The California Institute of Technology website.

[7] Ober C, Sinatra S, Zucker M. *Earthing: The Most Important Health Discovery Ever?* Laguna Beach, CA: Basic Health Publications, Inc.; 2010.

[8] Waterland RA, Jirtle RL. Early nutrition, epigenetic changes at transposons and imprinted genes, and enhanced susceptibility to adult chronic diseases. *Nutrition.* 2004; 20(1): 63-68.

[9] Fallon S, Enig MG. Guts and Grease: The Diet of Native Americans. The Weston A. Price Foundation website. Published January 1 2000. Accessed January 2017.

[10] Roach M. *Gulp: Adventures on the Alimentary Canal.* New York, NY: W.W. Norton and Company, Inc.; 2013.

[11] Alavanja MCR. Pesticides use and exposure extensive worldwide. *Reviews on Environmental Health.* 2009;24(4):303-309.

[12] Russo GL. Dietary n-6 and n-3 polyunsaturated fatty acids: from biochemistry to clinical implications in cardiovascular prevention. *Biochem Pharmacol.* 2009;77(6): 937-46.

[13] Barclay E. Your grandparents spent more of their money on food than you do. *National Public Radio.* March 2 2015.

[14] Teicholz N. *The Big Fat Surprise: Why Butter, Meat and Cheese Belong in a Healthy Diet.* New York, NY: Simon and Schuster Paperbacks; 2014.

[15] Clayton P, Rowbotham J. How mid-Victorians worked, ate and died. *Int. J. Environ. Res. Public Health.* 2009; 6(3): 1235-1253.

[16] Ferrières J. The French paradox: lessons for other countries. *Heart.* 2004;90(1):107-111.

[17] Kell J. Lean times for the diet industry. *Fortune.* May 21 2015.

[18] Libby P. Inflammation and cardiovascular disease mechanisms. *Am J Clin Nutr.* 2006; 83(2): 4565-4605.

[19] Russo GL. Dietary n-6 and n-3 polyunsaturated fatty acids: from biochemistry to clinical implications in cardiovascular prevention. *Biochem Pharmacol.* 2009;77(6): 937-46.

[20] Pollack GH. *The Fourth Phase of Water: Beyond Solid, Liquid and Vapor.* Seattle, WA: Ebner and Sons Publishing; 2013.

[21] Montagnier L, Aïssa J, Ferris S, Montagnier JL, Lavallée C. Electromagnetic signals are produced by aqueous nanostructures derived from bacterial DNA sequences. *Interdisciplinary Sciences, Computational Life Sciences.* 2009; 1(2): 81–90.

[22] Levine JA. What are the risks of sitting too much? Mayo Clinic website. Published September 4 2015.

[23] Ergotron JustStand® Survey & Index Report. Ergotron website. 2013

[24] Young DR, Reynolds K, Sidell M, et al. Effects of physical activity and sedentary time on the risk of heart failure. *Circulation: Heart Failure.* 2014; 7(1): 21-27.

[25] Owen N, Healy GN, Matthews CE, and Dunstan DW. Too much sitting: the population-health science of sedentary behavior. *Exerc Sport Sci Rev.* 2010; 38(3): 105–113.

[26] Warren TY, Barry V, Hooker SP, Sui X, Church TS, Blair SN. Sedentary behaviors increase risk of cardiovascular disease mortality in men. *Med Sci Sports Exerc.* 2010; 42(5): 879-85.

[27] Vernikos J. *Sitting Kills, Moving Heals.* Fresno, CA: Quill Driver Books; 2011.

[28] Levine JA. Non-exercise activity thermogenesis (NEAT). *Best Pract Res Clin Endocrinol Metab.* 2002; 16(4): 679-702.

[29] Boutcher SH. High-Intensity Intermittent Exercise and Fat Loss. *Journal of Obesity.* 2011.

[30] International Agency for Research on Cancer. IARC classifies radiofrequency electromagnetic fields as possibly carcinogenic to humans. World Health Organization website. Published May 31 2011.

[31] Fields RD. Mind control by cellphone. *Scientific American.* May 7 2008.

[32] Electromagnetic and radiofrequency fields effect on human health. American Academy of Environmental Medicine website.

[33] National Center for Health Statistics. National Health and Nutrition Examination Survey. Centers for Disease Control and Prevention website. Last updated May 30 2017.

[34] How much is too much?: Appendix b: vitamin and mineral deficiencies in the U.S. Environmental Working Group website. Published June 19 2014.

Further Reading

The Fourth Phase of Water: Beyond Solid, Liquid, and Vapor by Gerald H. Pollack

The Disease Delusion: Conquering the Causes of Chronic Illness for a Healthier, Longer and Happier Life by Jeffrey Bland

Secrets of Your Cells: Discovering Your Body's Inner Intelligence by Sondra Barret, PhD

Earthing: The Most Important Health Discovery Ever? by Clinton Ober, Stephen T. Sinatra, M.D., and Martin Zucker

Food Rules: An Eater's Manual by Michael Pollan

Fat as Fuel: A Revolutionary Diet to Combat Cancer, Boost Brain Power, and Increase Your Energy by Joseph Mercola

Sitting Kills, Moving Heals: How Everyday Movement Will Prevent Pain, Illness, and Early Death—and Exercise Won't by Joan Vernikos

Acknowledgments

This book could not have happened without the amazing help of my wife, Laurie McQuaig, D.C., and a dear friend, Amie Forest, Creative Director of Forest Design LLC. Both of them helped tremendously in getting "the project done," and together were a creative force. They were full of ideas and endless rewrites and kept me going when I wanted to quit. It was as if a gift I never expected landed in my lap. I actually enjoyed the process. Amie created the cover design. My wife, Laurie, has also been the other half of the Seattle Natural Health (SNH) doctor team from the beginning. She is a true healer and has helped transform many lives.

Additionally, I want to thank another dear friend, Karl Forest, who helped with editing in a number of chapters. Thank you to my children, Peter and Lise, who were endlessly optimistic and encouraging as they read and commented from Walla Walla, Washington and Seville, Spain. Much appreciation goes out to my family and friends who have been so supportive and sources of inspiration to me.

My deepest gratitude goes out to current and former staff members at SNH. For the last two decades plus, you all have always shown up ready to help improve the health and vitality of everyone who comes through our doors. We have shared many laughs, tears and long days together.

Having you in the clinic has enriched the patients' and my experience. You have been great to put up with my quirks and crazy early morning schedule. The success of SNH has come from all of us. Each of you has a spot in my heart full of gratitude and love. Thank you so much.

Of course none of this could have happened without my parents. They loved me unconditionally and always encouraged me to be the very best and loving human being possible. Although they are no longer here, I know they would have been cheering me on to write this book. I feel as though a part of them is in these words.

To my brothers, Lee and John, thank you for teaching me the meaning of play and the essentials of this book: barefoot in the backyard out in the sun for hours on end.

I would like to acknowledge the works of Dr. Pollack, PhD for his research on water and Jack Kruse, M.D., who helps blend the best of science and our humanness to improve our health. I want to thank my mentors Dr. George Goodheart, Dr. Wally Schmitt, Dr. Jeffrey Bland and Dr. John Brimhall for teaching me so much about healing and being the best clinician possible.

Thanks also to editor Maggie McReynolds and Angela Lauria. I appreciate your work.

Most of all I would like to acknowledge the patients

who have blessed me over the years. I have learned so much from each and every one of you, and I feel that it is a privilege to be a part of your lives. This book and journey could not have happened without you. You have touched my life in so many ways. I am so grateful to you all.

About the Author

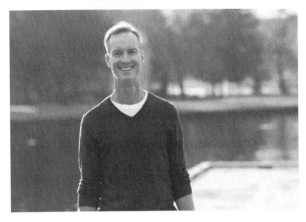

Dr. David Ramaley has spent the last 24 years helping people achieve incredible health and vitality. As a naturopath and chiropractor, he incorporates natural approaches with the latest scientific research. He attended Bastyr University and Life Chiropractic College West, and received a Diplomate in Chiropractic Neurology. He co-founded Seattle Natural Health, LLC., a clinic that focuses on acute and chronic health issues and solutions to those problems.

Dr. Ramaley is a writer, lecturer, and educator on health and nutrition. He is an innovative thinker, is passionate about health and human performance, and thrives on helping people resolve health challenges. He lives in Seattle with his wife, also a chiropractor. They have a son and daughter who make great playmates and pursue their own passions. Dr. Ramaley also loves to exercise, spend time outdoors, make fermented foods and shop at the farmers market.

drramaley.com | info@drramaley.com | facebook.com/DrDavidRamaley